HOW TO Stay Sane IN Your Baby's First Year

This book belongs to:
Yeovil, Sherborne & District NCT
When you have finished reading it please return to:
Donna Banfield
01963 371 651

(and me!)

All my love,

Alan

xxx

HOW TO Stay Sane IN Your Baby's First Year

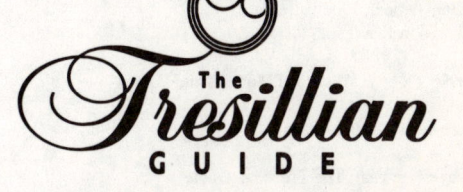

The Tresillian Guide

REVISED EDITION

Cathrine Fowler & Patricia Gornall

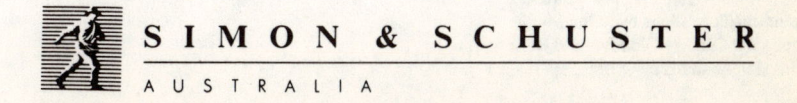

SIMON & SCHUSTER
AUSTRALIA

HOW TO STAY SANE IN YOUR BABY'S FIRST YEAR: THE TRESILLIAN GUIDE
REVISED EDITION
First published in Australasia in 1991 by
Simon & Schuster Australia
20 Barcoo Street, East Roseville NSW 2069

A Viacom Company
Sydney New York London Toronto Tokyo Singapore

Reprinted in 1991, 1992, 1993 (twice), 1994
Revised edition first published in 1996
Reprinted in 1996
© 1991 and 1996 Royal Society for the Welfare of Mothers and Babies
  Tresillian Family Care Centres
  Catherine Fowler and Patricia Gornall
  Fowler, Catherine
  How to stay sane in baby's first year: The Tresillian Guide

  Rev. ed
  Includes index.
  ISBN 0 7318 0651 4

  1. Infants - care. I. Gornall, Patricia. II. Title

649.122

All rights reserved. No part of this publication may be reproduced, sorted in a retrieval system, or transmitted, in any form or by any means, electronic, mechanical, photocopying, recording or otherwise, without the prior permission of the publisher in writing.

Edited by Maro Lanagan
Design Steven Dunbar
Revised edition formatted by Joy Eckermann
Cartoon illustrations by Jack Newnham
Technical illustrations by Robin Mudie
Typeset in Century Old Style and Helvetica
Printed in Australia by Griffin Paperbacks

Foreword

One of the most important conversations of my life occurred in November 1983 with an Infant Health Centre sister, shortly after the birth of my daughter, Eliza.

I had fronted up for one of my early visits as a new mum. I was a 'career' woman, with just over ten years in the work force, and expected to be relatively capable of meeting a variety of challenges. Most, that is, except the challenge of a new little person, for which all my professional experience seemed useless.

This nurse took charge immediately. With gruff aplomb, she proceeded to check out baby and mother and then dispense what I still consider to be the best single piece of parenting advice I've ever had: 'If you answer her basic needs, she will learn to trust you first, then she'll learn to trust herself. And that is the secret of character development,' she proclaimed. Simple. Understandable. True.

I hung on to that because it sounded so right, as did another friend's wise, gentle remark: 'Do, above all, what you think is right.'

Both cut through all the platitudes and conflicting advice, all the fashions and fads. Both encouraged me to develop my own way of being a parent and to develop my own confidence. I was a bit tottery at the start, as is everyone at the beginning of a new adventure, but I gradually learned and I'm still practising!

But one never quite 'arrives' as a parent, in an absolute sense. It is one of life's great explorations, with pots of gold dotted along a path for which the map is sometimes rather problematic.

This book, produced by the exceptionally useful Tresillian Family Care Centres, helps in a way many books don't with that vital first year. I love the way it provides actual, practical advice, as well as theory. For instance, I particularly appreciated chapter 3, 'Survival techniques for parents'. It gives hints about quick relaxation techniques, about using a nappy service or disposables for at least the first month. It says sensible things about establishing vital priorities in housework, reducing it, maybe, to only making your bed and keeping the lounge room tidy, and setting aside one night a week when you and your partner will *definitely* have takeaway food. This is all so eminently reasonable and do-able. But it's good to see it written down like that, because it instantly encourages the new parents to consider new ways of doing things.

The notion that the baby will make no difference to your life is nonsense! The sooner couples acknowledge that and get on with the business of jointly planning a new home pattern, the better.

The earlier the changes, the earlier you'll become expert at flexibility, the more you'll realise that anything is possible with a baby—it just takes a little longer and you may not be able to achieve it all in one day. But after one year, you'll be astonished at how efficient you become.

This book offers optimism because it gives practical advice, and that's what new parents need most. I heartily recommend that all prospective grandparents buy one for their offspring . . . and read it themselves too. Real mothers, fathers and babies are discussed, not theories and models of perfection: therein happy children do not lie, that much I am sure of.

Geraldine Doogue
Sydney 1991

Contents

Foreword 5
President's note 8
Introduction 9
Contact numbers 14

You
1 Preparing for your baby 16
2 After your baby arrives 34
3 Survival techniques for parents 54
4 Coping with crying and lack of sleep 63
5 Post-natal depression 78

Your baby
6 From birth to three months 85
7 From three months to six months 101
8 From six months to nine months 108
9 From nine months to one year 116

Feeding your baby
10 Breastfeeding 126
11 Common breastfeeding problems 141
12 Weaning 151
13 Bottlefeeding 159
14 The introduction of solids 171
15 Recipes 184

Special situations
16 Travelling with your baby 192
17 Caring for your sick baby 203
18 Leaving your baby in care 219

Appendices
I Safety 226
II Support services—Australia and New Zealand 241
III Immunisation schedules 251
IV Emergency treatment 254

Index 259
Acknowledgements 264

President's note

The Council of Tresillian congratulate the authors of *How to Stay Sane in Your Baby's First Year*. The authors are Cathrine Fowler, Manager of our Education Department (also holder of the Public Service Medal for services to NSW Health and Tresillian Family Care Centres), and Patricia Gornall, Senior Nurse Educator. First published in 1991, the success of the book has been such as to warrant this second edition. It is following in the footsteps of an earlier Tresillian publication entitled *Parent's Book*, of which there were nineteen editions.

The book admirably achieves the purpose of conveying information to parents in simple, intelligible terms, well illustrated, to help them enjoy the experience of parenting. It thus blends in well with Tresillian's mission, which is 'to promote the health and wellbeing of families with babies and young children'. Furthermore, the book neatly complements the advice given by Tresillian staff at the Family Care Centres and on the Parent Help Line. We are proud of this book and we believe it will continue to be one of the top parenting books in Australia.

Bob Elmslie
PRESIDENT

Introduction

The Royal Society for the Welfare of Mothers and Babies, now commonly called Tresillian Family Care Centres, was formed in 1918 to co-ordinate early childhood and maternal services in New South Wales.

The society was formed in response to the high death rate of children under the age of five years. During the First World War about 63 000 Australian servicemen lost their lives fighting overseas, while in Australia about 70 000 children under the age of five lost their lives through poverty, disease and lack of hygiene.

Tresillian initially responded to the problem at home with a community education programme for parents of small children. Its other aims were:

> To Save Baby Life.
> To co-ordinate all existing Agencies for dealing with Mothers and Babies.
> To ensure proper Nursing Conditions to every mother prior and subsequent to Childbirth.
> To establish Welfare Centres and Committees in the Metropolis and Country.
> To establish Rest Homes for Mothers.
> To establish a Corps of Mothers' Aids.
> To care for and bring under supervision all Children up to school age.
> To provide certified and Humanised Milk, and Ice.
> *Annual Report* 1920–21

In 1921 the first hospital, 'Tresillian', was started at Shaw Street, Petersham, in Sydney. Dr Margaret Harper, the first medical director, established a school at the hospital to educate baby health centre sisters, to work with parents to address some of the basic problems of lack of hygiene, and to carry out immunisation programmes.

Tresillian's tradition of education has continued over the years. Courses for both professionals and parents are offered still through Tresillian Family Care Centres, but the emphasis has changed from disease prevention and infant survival to health promotion and meeting the changing needs of parents.

Services offered to parents include a 24-hour Parent Help Line, which is utilised by parents throughout Australia and occasionally from overseas. In 1994, 64000 calls were taken. This service offers practical parenting advice as well as emotional support for parents with small children, and refers parents to other community services.

The Outreach Service is an innovative family health service that offers a home visiting service to parents on the lower North Shore of Sydney and in the inner western suburbs.

The Day Stay Clinics at Petersham, Wollstonecraft and Penrith cater for parents needing professional assistance with problems of various kinds. These range from breastfeeding and bottlefeeding difficulties to coping with toddler behaviour.

Emergency occasional care operates at the Wollstonecraft day-stay unit and provides time out for parents who need it.

The residential units at Petersham, Willoughby and Penrith have established a solid reputation for providing parents who live in with support and 24-hour professional advice about themselves, their babies and their toddlers. The Willoughby and Penrith units have a special unit for toddler management and advice.

The Guthrie Child Care Centre offers long day care services for children (up to the age of five) of disadvantaged parents.

The Tresillian post-natal depression service offers counselling, management and support to parents with post-natal depression. The health care team offers ongoing professional and community education and is conducting research into the many and varied aspects of parenting crises and post-natal depression.

Tresillian's philosophy is one of supporting parents in their new roles and encouraging them to make informed decisions and to follow the parenting style of their choice. The support that Tresillian gives

INTRODUCTION

helps parents enjoy their new roles and their new baby.

Today society places many pressures on parents. There have been marked changes in the expectations the community has of both men and women in the parenting role, as well as the expectations new parents themselves have of parenting. The effects of these changes have been intensified by the mobility of the population, which has isolated many new parents from their immediate families and support people.

Once, parents received support, practical assistance and basic child-rearing advice from their immediate families, and often gained some experience of caring for children by looking after their siblings. The trend towards smaller families, the greater integration of women into the paid work force, and the increasing belief that fathers should provide practical as well as financial assistance in the rearing of their children, have all contributed to parental anxiety.

In this book we have tried to give information that is often difficult to find; for example, on weaning. Many books discuss breast-feeding or the introduction of solids, but rarely do they provide practical advice on how to wean. We have also included basic information that might once have been handed down from parent to child, but which may not be as generally known these days.

The term 'early childhood health nurse' has been used throughout this book. Early childhood health nurses are educated specifically in parenting issues and the care of babies and children up to the age of five years (in some states, up to eighteen years). The majority have nursing qualifications in general, midwifery and child and family health nursing, as well as counselling and support expertise. Their titles vary across Australia from early childhood health nurses to child health nurses, community health nurses, infant health nurses, and maternal and child health nurses. In New Zealand they are called Plunket nurses. They can be a great help and support to you in your new parenting role.

THE TRESILLIAN GUIDE

Parenting can be difficult. For all parents at some time it is an entirely new experience. The quantity and variety of advice available, and the fact that it is often conflicting, do not make the experience any easier. This book will provide basic, clear guidelines for you to follow in caring for yourself and your baby.

Use this information in your decision-making about the care of your child. With every day that passes, your confidence will increase and you will start to enjoy your baby more and settle into your new role as a parent.

In this book we offer some practical solutions to common problems. We also hope that you will remember that each day is a new day, and that maintaining a sense of humour will greatly help you in enjoying this time of your lives.

We have deliberately made this book directive in parts for two reasons. Firstly, when you are new to any experience, whether driving a car or caring for a baby, it is handy to have specific advice to follow. If you ask an experienced cook to tell you how she makes a certain dish, she might say 'Oh, I don't follow a recipe. I just put in a bit of this and a bit of that and then judge by the look of the mixture', which is not a lot of help if you want to cook the dish yourself! If you ask for advice regarding baby care from your parents or others who are familiar with small babies, you often get a similar response. Later you will know how to do these things without effort and be able to think about other things while you do them, but at the beginning, you may need detailed direction and explanations.

Secondly, there are many fads in parenting; different techniques are always going in and out of fashion. In the 1950s and 1960s, feeding your baby every four hours was in vogue, for instance, and during the 1980s there was a fashion for feeding whenever the baby cried. The pendulum has now swung back to a point between these two extremes, and many parents feed with a certain amount of routine but remain flexible.

We have tried in this book to give you the basics of parenting advice,

INTRODUCTION

and to ignore as much as possible the fads that come and go with the seasons.

It will be up to you to decide what is best for you and your baby. Do not limit your options; listen to and assess any advice you are given or that you read, and do whatever works for you. The bottom line is that you, your partner and your baby are well and happy.

THE TRESILLIAN GUIDE

Contact numbers

Photocopy this page and place it on the refrigerator or by the telephone.

Ambulance/Fire/Police: **000 (111 in New Zealand)**

Nearest cross street:

Poisons Information Service 13 1126 (Australia wide)

Local Police Station:

Doctor:

Local hospital:

Early childhood health nurse:

Tresillian 24-hour Parent Help Line: (02) 569 5400 — 1 800 637 357 (NSW and ACT only)

Chemist:

Support people:

Neighbour:

Occasional care:

Other important contact numbers:

You

CHAPTER 1

Preparing for your baby

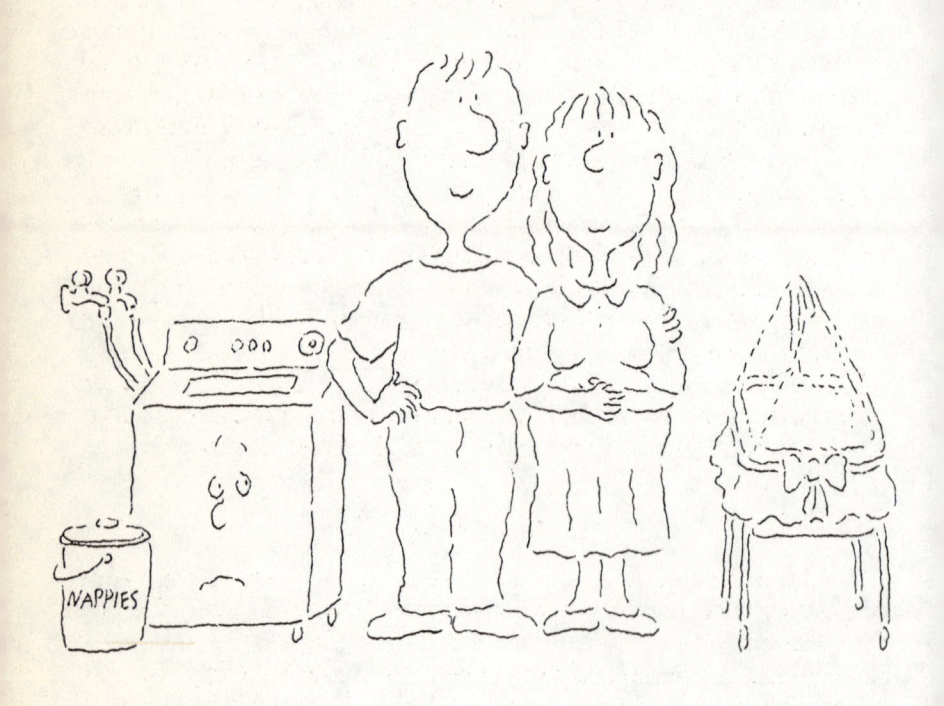

Preparing for the arrival of a baby is not, of course, simply a matter of obtaining the right equipment. The transition from being a reasonably freewheeling single person, or one half of a couple, to becoming a parent is a major step in any person's life, and sometimes can be as difficult as it is rewarding.

Planning begins before the birth, and even, for some parents-to-be, before conception. There are many significant decisions you should make well in advance, and if you are in a relationship, these will probably have to be made after a great deal of discussion and negotiation. For most couples the choices regarding working arrangements and childcare are becoming necessary. You should consider them in plenty of time to make such arrangements as applying for maternity and/or paternity leave and choosing a childcare centre.

The birth you want

Another decision that must be made early in the pregnancy concerns the type of birth you wish to have. You may want a birth at a hospital, or you may want a home birth with a midwife and a couple of support people present. Your choice will depend on the facilities in your area, such as the availability of midwives or birth centres, as much as on your personal preferences. You should investigate all possibilities thoroughly.

If both parents are going to be present, it will be a more rewarding experience if each is equally well informed regarding the birth process and the roles each is to play. Make sure that everyone who is going to be present at the birth is very clear as to the reasons for all your choices, so that at the time of the birth you can retain control of the situation, if that is what you wish. Also, build some degree of flexibility into your birth plan, so that if, for example, there are complications involved in your planned home birth, a transfer to hospital can be made smoothly, without confusion and without either parent feeling disappointed or guilty.

Classes

Your doctor, midwife or obstetrician will be guiding you through your pregnancy with advice appropriate to every stage, and there are many books available about pregnancy and childbirth. Childbirth education or preparation-for-parenthood classes may also be available in your area during the day or in the evening, run by hospitals, early childhood health centres or community health centres, or by private organisations. Most of these encourage the attendance of the pregnant woman's partner or support person, and they can be a great form of support for prospective parents. Most classes are very popular, so book in early.

Such classes usually involve a significant component of health education, advising parents-to-be on appropriate exercises, diet and safe remedies for minor ailments encountered during pregnancy. Many pregnancy manuals cover similar ground.

Ultrasound scan

There are a number of tests that will be done in the course of the pregnancy to monitor the mother's health and to determine whether the baby is developing normally. Among these will probably be an ultrasound scan, in which soundwaves are passed through the amniotic fluid in which the baby floats in the womb, using a hand-held instrument that is moved about on the surface of the stomach. This instrument receives the sound waves that are bounced off the developing baby, and an image is built up on a screen. In this way, problems of development can be detected at an early stage, as can multiple births and the position of the baby and placenta.

The scan can be uncomfortable if carried out in the early stages of pregnancy, as the mother must present for the scan with a full bladder so that her womb can be easily identified on the screen. Any discomfort will be compensated for by the thrill of seeing your baby for the first time; this can be a very exciting experience for fathers, too, as the reality of the baby is brought home.

Health hazards during pregnancy

All health professionals will advise against smoking (including passive smoking) during pregnancy and in a household in which there is a new baby. If either parent smokes, giving up is going to be easier early in the pregnancy than in the early weeks after the birth, when you will both be under stress from your new roles. There is now a great deal of evidence to support the claim that smoking during pregnancy affects the size of the baby, and that passive smoking has definite harmful effects on infants. The incidence of respiratory diseases such as asthma is increased if one parent smokes, and chemicals from cigarette smoking can be transferred to your baby through breastmilk.

If you give up smoking during the pregnancy, but take it up again after your baby is born, don't smoke in the car or in the same room as him, and insist that visitors who smoke do so in a room away from him. This is especially necessary in the first year of your baby's life, when he cannot move away from cigarette smoke and therefore becomes an involuntary smoker—increasing his risk of Sudden Infant Death Syndrome.

Drinking alcohol is similarly advised against for pregnant women, as the drug can cross the placental barrier and affect the growth of your baby's vital organs. If you cannot cut alcohol out entirely, it is better to drink only a very small amount at a time, rather than going for a spell without it and then drinking to excess.

Any form of medication a pregnant woman needs to take should be prescribed by a health professional who has taken her pregnancy into account. Always make sure you know about the possible side-effects of any medication you take at this crucial time, so that you can make an informed decision as to whether to take it.

First aid

To help you feel competent as a parent in a practical way, it is useful, before the baby arrives, to take first aid classes so that you will be prepared to deal with accidents and other emergencies. Organisations such as the Red Cross Society and St John Ambulance Association hold classes, often in the evenings so that you can attend if you work during the day. If you do not have a first aid kit, you can buy one from a first aid association in your state or from your local chemist or hardware store, or make up your own from the directions on page 226. If you have one already, it is a good idea to add some Syrup of Ipecac and some infant paracetamol before the birth. This is particularly necessary if you live in an area frequently isolated by the weather. If you do not have ready access to medical help, be sure that all the contact phone numbers you might need in an emergency are readily to hand before leaving hospital.

Adopting a baby

If you are adopting a baby, similar kinds of practical arrangements for his arrival will be necessary and, like any new parents, you should be prepared for the presence of a baby in your household to make major and sometimes unexpected changes in your lives. It is likely that the initial adjustments will have to be made quite rapidly, as the long wait for your baby may end suddenly when a child becomes available. You may be required to travel, with little advance warning, to the nearest city or even overseas to collect your new baby, and one parent may have to give up work quite abruptly and become a carer and houseworker. You will need time to get to know your baby, and may feel that being a parent is not as you expected it would be. These are normal feelings. Take time to adjust, and do not expect too much of yourself. If you are feeling overwhelmed or angry with your baby, talk to someone sympathetic about your feelings.

Isolation

Isolation is not just a problem for people who live in remote areas. Even in the most crowded of cities, new parents can find themselves trapped in a home unit, block of flats or caravan with the baby and no one to talk to. There is no longer the automatic support that was once provided by the structure of the extended family; new parents are often geographically isolated from their own parents. This can happen to people who have perhaps worked outside the home before the baby came along, or who, because of their partner's employment or for some other reason, have moved away from family members and friends. You may be lucky enough to have sympathetic friends who are going through parenthood themselves. If you do not, you may find that friends without children can no longer identify with you the way they used to. Because of this, it is important *before* you have your baby to devote some energy to constructing a network of support for yourself as a parent.

This may be simply a matter of listing the telephone numbers of organisations you can call on in an emergency, such as hospitals, early childhood centres and so on. Other people who attend your antenatal classes can be helpful and reassuring contacts also, and can become friends as your children grow up together. Any group or class that you join in your area will put you in touch with local people who can provide company or conversation—not necessarily about new babies!—when you are feeling lonely or fed up. If you cannot drive, it is worthwhile learning, as the use of a car will greatly decrease your isolation.

For other advice on combating isolation, see the section on 'Keeping in touch' on page 59.

Childproofing

Childproofing your house is another practical thing to do before the baby arrives; childproofing by trial and error can be hair-raising.

It is common for new parents to move house just before or soon after the arrival of their baby; they may feel that they need a bigger house to accommodate a child, or a house without stairs, or a backyard for the baby to play in, or a house closer to their relatives. Whatever the reason, it's not a good idea to move during the few months before and after the birth. Moving house takes a lot of emotional and physical energy that, added to the pressures of having a new baby, can be too much for parents to cope with.

If your home or unit is small, be creative with the placement of your furniture, and use screens or curtains to section off areas if you are all living in the one room. To begin with, you may not need a separate room for your new baby; many parents prefer to have the baby sleep in their room for the first few months. If you already have a toddler, and she does not have problems sleeping, she may like the idea of sharing her room with the new baby; this can help develop a close, caring relationship between siblings.

Before the baby arrives, look at ways of short-cutting housework. Keep bench-tops clear so that they are always easy to clean. Put away ornaments that collect dust. Consider using a continental quilt in the winter months, rather than sheets and blankets. Adequate storage facilities in the home are probably the greatest time savers; uncluttered surfaces are easier to clean and will be much safer when your baby reaches the exploring stage. Sit on the floor in each room and check the room for potential danger spots that need attention. A safe environment for your baby means that you won't need to be constantly saying 'Don't touch!' and 'No!' to him.

Use appendix I as a guide to childproofing your home.

Preparing your older child

If you have a toddler, make sure you prepare her for the arrival of the new baby, so that her feelings of rivalry with her sibling are minimised. Try to put yourself in her shoes. It is difficult for a toddler to cope with suddenly having to share you. As parents your time will be even more limited than previously, and you will need to be careful that your toddler does not become jealous, which can result in temper tantrums and clinging behaviour.

Before your baby is born, involve the toddler in as many aspects of the preparation as you can. (Remember that toddlers have very poor concepts of time—don't tell her about the new baby the minute you have your pregnancy confirmed, or you will have to put up with eight months of constant nagging!) Have her help with the setting up of the nursery. Read her books that deal with the arrival of new babies, and visit friends who have small babies if you can. Give your toddler some small role to play so that she feels useful and helpful. If you are having your toddler minded at someone else's house, have her stay there overnight on a 'holiday', to get used to the idea.

When you go into labour, if you are going to a hospital, wake your toddler and tell her you are going. Don't sneak out, even if you have to wake her at three in the morning. It is better having her know when and why you are going, even if it makes her cry, than her finding you gone in the morning. Sleep problems can occur later if she is worried that you might disappear unexpectedly during the night. A visit to the hospital with you before the birth will help her become familiar with the hospital environment.

Have her visit you while you are in hospital. She may be upset when she has to leave, but it is important that she can see that you are safe and well. Remember, she is still small and will need time to adjust to the baby.

Circumcision

The decision as to whether you will have your son circumcised is best made before he arrives. Circumcision involves the removal of part of the foreskin of the penis, and used to be carried out without the use of an anaesthetic while the mother and baby were in hospital.

The purpose of the foreskin is to protect the penis from damage and irritation. There is a very slight risk that uncircumcised boys will develop an infection under the foreskin, but in most cases this can be prevented by good hygiene, and the risk is outweighed by the risks of haemorrhage and infection arising from the circumcision operation. In Australia in recent years circumcision has been discouraged except for religious and medical reasons, and most small boys are now uncircumcised. A common reason for circumcision is to make the son look like the father, but most children will be more concerned about not looking like their peers. Parents who wish to have their son circumcised are encouraged to wait until he is at least six months old and ideally until he is out of nappies, when the operation should be performed by a paediatric surgeon using a general anaesthetic.

Baby care equipment

It's easy to be daunted by the range of baby care products on the market, and the considerable cash outlay that seems to be necessary even before your baby arrives. The two most common traps for new parents to fall into are the 'wait-and-see' attitude, which results in frazzled new parents making emergency shopping trips for nappies and nursery furniture as the need becomes evident, and the 'model-consumer' attitude, which sees the nursery fully outfitted and decorated in the early months of pregnancy.

The most sensible attitude to take, of course, lies somewhere between these two extremes. Don't rush out and buy everything you think you might possibly need early in the pregnancy. You will probably find that friends and relatives have spare rooms cluttered with disused strollers, cots, bassinettes and bouncers, not to mention bags of stored baby clothes and cot linen, which they will be only too happy to lend or give to you. On the other hand, it's nice to have a few things that you have bought or made specially for your baby. Some things, such as mattresses, nappy-changing accessories and dummies, should be bought new for every baby.

It's important to be as aware as possible of the types of equipment available. If older relatives offer to buy some major piece of equipment, such as a cot, they may have in mind something that was fashionable in their day, but is now regarded as unsafe. On the other hand, many modern features of baby care equipment are simply gimmicks, and as a parent and a consumer it is up to you to learn to identify quality products. In this section we have tried to cater for parents whose resources may be limited, and for whom the addition of another small human being to the household may strain an already tight budget. At the same time, we have tried not to omit extra products that might make life a little easier when the baby arrives.

Setting up the nursery

Setting up your baby's nursery can be very expensive. The important thing to remember is that babies don't know whether their equipment is secondhand, borrowed or brand new. The majority of baby furniture has a very limited period of use, dependent on the size and activity of your baby as he grows, and this factor should be taken into account when you are considering major purchases. You should also make sure that every piece of equipment is safe, and that it is easy to clean.

The basic piece of equipment for a nursery is a place for your baby to sleep. You may wish to buy a cot straight away, but for the first few months you may prefer something smaller—a bassinette or a carry-cot, for example. While you may be tempted to allow your baby to sleep in his pram or capsule, this is not recommended as a general practice, as most prams or capsules do not provide sufficient ventilation or support.

One thing to watch for if you are buying a secondhand cot, or have received an old one as a gift, is the type of paint it is covered with. If the paint contains lead there is a definite risk of poisoning if, in the teething stages, your baby chews some paint off and swallows it. Stripping all the paint off and repainting or varnishing will be necessary.

Any catch that allows you to raise and lower the sides of the cot should be easy to operate with one hand while you hold the baby, but not so easy as to allow the baby himself to undo it. Check also that it cannot trap a small finger.

Cots should conform to the Standards Association of Australia guidelines, including mattress size specifications. Bars should be between 5 and 8.5 cm (2–3 $\frac{1}{2}$") apart, and the whole cot should be sturdily built.

Carry cots have the advantage, of course, of being portable (though they are not recommended for use in cars—only an approved safety capsule should be used). They can be bought with wheeled bases or stands—if there are four wheels on the stand there should also be brakes or some way of immobilising the cot—and some can be attached to a wheeled frame and double as a pram. Cuddly Nests are not recommended because of the risk of overheating.

A **bassinette** should have a firm stand, with two wheels so that it can be moved about and rocked, and the base should be wide, for stability.

The **mattress** should be firm.

It is helpful to cover the lower half of the mattress in the cot or bassinette to protect it from soiling. You can buy cot- and bassinette-sized **mattress covers** with lengths of elastic that loop around the mattress. Commercial covers may not be available in the size you require, however, so you may prefer to make a cover yourself. Use a piece of heavy vinyl 30 cm (12") long (don't use light plastic such as that used for dry-cleaning bags, as there is a significant risk of suffocation involved), and cut it to the width of the mattress. Sew a length of cotton sheeting to each side edge of the vinyl to make it easier to tuck in. The vinyl should then be covered by the bottom sheet or a piece of sheeting cut to the same size as the vinyl. Instead of vinyl, you can use an old woollen blanket cut to size.

You will need three sets of cotton cot or bassinette **sheets**. These can be cut down from old full-sized cotton sheets: cut to the mattress size, leaving 20–26 cm (8–10") all around for tucking in. Always hem the material so that there are no loose threads for your baby's fingers or toes to become tangled in. Cot-sized sheets can be folded in half to fit a bassinette mattress.

Pillows should not be used with children under two years because of the danger of suffocation, but a **pillowcase**, or some other absorbent fabric between your baby's head and the sheet, can be a real time and energy saver, especially if your baby possets regularly or tends to have a sweaty head in hot weather. Leftover cotton sheeting is ideal, as is a lightweight summer nappy folded over the head end of the mattress.

Your baby will probably need a lightweight **blanket** in all but the height of summer. Tresillian advises a blanket made of a natural fibre—wool or cotton. If your baby or your family tends to suffer from skin complaints or allergies, invest in a cellular cotton blanket, which is less

PREPARING FOR YOUR BABY

likely to cause irritation to the skin and is easily washed. These are available in cot and bassinette sizes.

A **mosquito net** is a worthwhile investment to protect your baby from flying and biting insects. (Avoid spraying pesticides near your baby; flyscreens on windows and doors are worth considering.)

A **change table** is essential. This can be commercially made or be any large flat surface you feel comfortable changing your baby on. You should be able to leave it permanently set up for nappy changing. Make sure that it is stable and that the joints are secure and check that it is at a comfortable height so that you do not have to stoop to change your baby.

If you are not using a commercial change table, a **change mat** with padding along both sides and at the head end is advisable to keep your baby in position while you change him. A safety strap is essential to prevent him falling off the mat.

Within easy reach

When you are changing nappies, you will need to have the following articles close at hand:

- a small bottle of **surgical methylated spirits** with a tight-fitting lid, if advised by your maternity hospital. This is to clean your baby's umbilical cord, until it drops off and the umbilicus is healed. Make sure this is well out of reach of any other small children;

- **cotton tips** for applying the methylated spirits or, if your maternity hospital does not advise surgical methylated spirits, to dry the cord after the bath (don't use these to clean your baby's ears or nose, as they can cause damage);

- **nappies**, either in a folded stack or loose, to be folded as needed;

- **nappy liners**, either cloth or disposable, if you are using them;

- **nappy pins**, stored closed, if you are using them. If you want to avoid using pins, you can simply put a pilcher with adjustable fastening firmly over your baby's nappy—do not do this if your baby has sensitive skin or is currently suffering from nappy rash—or you can use shaped nappies with popper studs at the waist, which can save you a lot of folding but can be an expensive alternative. There are also self-fastening webbing-strap and clip arrangements that can be used to hold a nappy on;

- **cleaning agents and equipment for soiled bottoms.** This might be a bowl of warm water with soap, a washer and a towel, or a small container of olive oil or a commercial change lotion and cottonwool balls;

- **barrier cream**, such as zinc and castor oil, or petroleum jelly, to protect your baby's delicate buttock and groin area;
- **squares of old cotton cloth**, about 7 cm x 7 cm (3" x 3"), with which to apply creams. These help prevent contamination of creams with your fingers, solve the problem of continually getting creams under your fingernails, and when used as nappy liners, prevent the cream transferring itself to the nappy;
- a box of **tissues** to mop up spills;
- a brightly coloured **toy** to use as a distraction if your baby will not lie still or is upset. A musical toy is especially useful.

All the little things you need to care for your baby's skin and comfort at nappy-changing time can be stored in a **large plastic container** on the change table and readily transferred to a carry-bag when you go out.

A small **waste-basket**, lined with a plastic bag and preferably with a lid, is useful for discarding used tissues and cotton balls. It also helps to have **another plastic container** on hand for soiled nappies and clothes until you can take them to the laundry.

Feeding equipment

Whether or not you are planning to breastfeed, it is worthwhile having **a feeding bottle and a slow teat** (milk should drip through the hole at a rate of about one drop per second), in case you need to feed your baby expressed breastmilk, or bottlefeed him during an emergency. Sterilise the bottle before every use (see pages 164–5 for guidelilles) and clean it with a **bottle brush** afterwards.

If you are planning to bottlefeed your baby, chapter 13 (page 159) will help you decide what equipment you will need.

Dummies

A dummy can be a valuable piece of equipment, and is useful to have on hand for an emergency. It is advisable to use one only when you have tried other methods of settling or calming your baby. Once you have established that your baby will take a dummy, it is handy to have three dummies, so that you will always have a sterile dummy on hand if your baby drops one. Some babies are not at all interested in taking a dummy, and other methods can be used to settle them. If you do buy a dummy, purchase one that is approved by the Safety Standards of Australia.

Bathing equipment

A **baby bath** is a worthwhile investment, being more flexible and kinder to the parent's back than bathing a baby in a full-sized bath. When choosing a bath, make sure that it is deep enough for the baby to float and relax in it without becoming cold. When choosing a place in which to bath your baby, remember that it should be out of draughts, close to a sink or tub with hot and cold water (you should never carry a bath full of water, but should use a jug or small bucket to fill the bath, to avoid straining your back), and at a comfortable height so that you do not have to stoop to hold the baby. If the floor is slippery you will need to wipe up spilled water straight away to lessen the danger of you slipping over, and you might have to put down a firmly anchored mat in your chosen bathing place.

You will need a soft **towel** large enough to wrap up the baby securely. You should keep one towel especially for your baby's use when he is very young, for the sake of hygiene and cleanliness.

Some parents like to have two **washers**, one to use on the baby's face and one for the rest of his body.

Avoid using perfumed **soaps**, as they can cause irritation to your baby's sensitive skin. If you want to soap him, keep a non-perfumed cake of soap for his exclusive use.

If you are going to massage your baby after his bath, have the necessary **oil** to hand. The olive oil you use for cooking is perfectly suitable for massage. Other unperfumed organic oils such as almond, jojoba, wheatgerm or apricot are suitable also. Commercial baby oils often contain mineral oils, which are actually drying for your baby's skin.

Laundry equipment

Unless you are lucky enough to have the permanent use of a nappy wash and laundry service, a **washing machine** is indispensable in a household with a new baby. If you are planning a winter baby, access to a **clothes dryer** is helpful if your home is too small to allow you to hang up a great deal of wet washing indoors.

You will need a large **bucket with a lid** to soak nappies in. Make sure the lid fits tightly, so that a small child would find it impossible to remove. If you can, keep it out of the reach of small children, perhaps placing it in the laundry trough.

If you are using the soaking method to clean your nappies (see page 94), buy a trial pack of **commercial nappy-cleaning solution or powder** to start you off. Store it out of reach of small children. If you are using the washing-machine method, have a packet of **pure soap powder** on hand.

Additional equipment

There are a multitude of makes and models, from basic to deluxe, of **prams and strollers** and combinations of the two. If you are buying a new one for your baby, look for the following features. It should:

- have functioning brakes that will hold on a steep incline;
- be well balanced and easy to push, including up and down stairs and onto and off gutters; the larger the wheels, the more manoeuvrable the pram. These first two requirements can be difficult to test in a shop—if possible, try out friends' prams and strollers to help you decide;
- be easy to clean; all fabric that is not removable and machine washable should be able to be sponged clean;
- be compact and foldable to a manageable size. This is especially important if you are going to be limited to public transport, particularly buses;
- be adjustable, so that your baby can lie flat in it while very young and be sat up in it as he grows;
- have no dangerous sharp edges;
- have a good-sized hood to protect the baby from the sun;
- have a built-in basket or shelf on which to carry shopping and a baby bag; and
- have handles high enough for you both to push it without stooping.

Many prams convert into strollers; when the baby is a little older this can save you the cost of a stroller.

As your baby becomes mobile, a **playpen** can be a useful piece of equipment, providing a safe space for your baby to play in if you are too busy to watch him for a little while, or saving older children from the frustration of having their play interrupted by a curious, wandering baby. Many parents set the playpen up around themselves while they iron or sew, as a safety precaution, leaving the baby to play outside the pen.

For similar reasons, **door barriers** in the form of low gates and fences are useful for keeping babies out of high-risk areas such as kitchens and stairways, without restricting their view of the action.

Many parents find **carry pouches** (for young babies, worn on the parent's front) and **backpacks** (for older babies with good head and back control) to be particularly useful. Babies can calm down quickly with the combination of body contact with a parent and the rhythmical motion of the parent's walking. Carry pouches and backpacks should be of simple construction and easy to put on and take off with or without the baby inside them. You should also make sure that the baby can be placed inside and taken out of the pouch or pack with the minimum of fuss. In a pouch, the baby's head and neck should be well supported and his arms and legs comfortable, without restricting his blood circulation.

Baby walkers have now been banned from sale because of the numerous accidents associated with their use.

Bouncinettes should also be used only for limited periods during the day. They are good for providing your baby with a change of position and environment. If you live in a very hot or humid region, a bouncinette covered with open-work stretch fabric allows air to flow around your baby's body and keep him cool. Take care to place the bouncinette on the floor rather than on a table or bench, as there is a real risk that your baby will bounce it off onto the floor. Always use the safety strap to hold your baby in the bouncinette.

Clothing

Most parents enjoy preparing the baby's clothing before a birth, trying to imagine how anyone's hand or foot could be so tiny. Friends and relatives are likely to provide both hand-me-downs and newly bought or knitted garments, so don't overbuy early in the pregnancy. Before your baby arrives, wash all the clothing he will be wearing in the first few weeks.

You will need two to three dozen **cloth nappies**. Buy heavyweight cotton with well-hemmed edges, as you will have to change your baby's nappy around 4500 times at a minimum. As an alternative, you can buy cloth nappies that are shaped to fit babies and adjustable as they grow; these will be more expensive, but will save you a lot of folding! Wash cloth nappies with pure soap powder before using them for the first time. **Disposable nappies** are great when travelling, or for when you run out of cloth nappies, but their 'disposability' is in question. If you use them, do not flush the nappy down the toilet. Remove as much heavy soiling from it as possible into the toilet. Then roll it into a bundle, use tapes to reseal and place it in a plastic bag before putting it in the garbage.

Protective pants or pilchers come in a variety of designs and fabrics. Whichever ones you prefer to use, make sure you have enough to change at frequent intervals. If pants are elasticised at the waist and around the tops of the legs, you will have to check when your baby arrives that the elastic is not too tight. Plastic pants are useful on outings but are not advisable for regular use, as they increase the risk of nappy rash developing.

You will probably need about six **singlets**. Unless you have a very small baby, size 00 or 0 will probably fit a newborn—the main difference in sizing appears to be the length rather than the width.

For **night wear**, you will probably need a minimum of six garments, either nighties or all-in-one jumpsuits, or a few of each. Nighties can be bought in a larger size and thus allow for growth; they are usually cooler in hot weather and they allow for easier nappy changing. All-in-one jumpsuits can be fiddly when you are changing your baby's nappy, especially at night, but have the advantage of keeping tiny toes warm, and don't roll up uncomfortably, as nighties have a tendency to do. They are easy to wash and need no ironing. Buy them with plenty of room for your baby's growing feet, and be prepared to cut them when your baby's feet grow. Jumpsuits with openings down the insides of both legs are advised, as they are easier to guide the baby's legs into.

You will need four **cardigans, jumpers or jackets**; the time of year and the climate will govern the style and weight you choose. Woollen jackets may irritate your baby's skin, so make sure he wears a softer fabric inside the jacket.

Because of the large surface area of his head, your baby can lose a great deal of heat if he does not wear a bonnet when taken outside on windy or cold days. You will probably only need two. A sunhat is necessary in the summer months to shade your baby's head and face.

Six pairs of **bootees or socks** is probably a reasonable number to have on hand. Often newborns are given bootees as gifts, so it may be wise to wait and see before buying them. Bootees or socks should be loose-fitting; the ankle ties should be made of ribbon rather than wool, as wool tends to stretch when it is being tied and then contract, constricting the baby's ankle. Loose-fitting socks work just as well as

PREPARING FOR YOUR BABY

EQUIPMENT CHECKLIST

NURSERY
Bassinette
Bassinette liner
Mattress—tea-tree filling with a cotton cover
Mattress cover
Sheets (3 sets)
Pillowcases (3)
Blanket—cotton or wool
Mosquito net
Change table or area set aside
Change mat
Surgical methylated spirits (if advised)
Cotton tips
Nappy liners
Nappy pins
Cleaning agents
Barrier cream—zinc and castor oil or petroleum jelly
Squares of cotton cloth
Box of tissues
Toy for distracting attention while nappy changing
Waste-basket
Plastic container for taking dirty nappies and clothing to the laundry
Dummy (1, to test whether a dummy settles your baby)

FEEDING EQUIPMENT
Feeding bottle with a slow teat
Bottle brush

BATHING EQUIPMENT
Baby bath
Towel
Washer(s)
Non-perfumed soap or other cleaning agent
Oil for massage

LAUNDRY EQUIPMENT
Washing machine
Nappy bucket with tightly fitting lid
Nappy sterilising solution or powder, or pure soap powder

OTHER EQUIPMENT
Safety capsule
Pram or stroller
Playpen
Door barrier(s)
Carry pouch or backpack

CLOTHING
Nappies (2–3 dozen)
Protective pants or pilchers
Singlets (6)
Nighties or jumpsuits (6)
Jackets, cardigans or jumpers (4)
Bonnets (2)
Bootees or socks (6 pairs)
Mittens (1 pair) in cold areas
Cuddlies or baby blankets (4)
Towelling bibs (6)

bootees, and are usually easier to wash. Always check the insides of bootees and socks for loose threads, as these can cause grave injury if they wind around your baby's toes.

Mittens will only be needed if you live in a very cold area. Mittens should always be made of cotton fabric, not knitted or crocheted, to reduce the risk of his fingers becoming caught in the fabric. French (concealed) seams should be used to protect your baby's fingers from loose threads. Check your baby's fingers at each nappy change in case they have become tangled or constricted in any way.

Cuddlies or baby rugs are essential, as babies like to be wrapped or swaddled in the early months. Cuddlies should be made of a washable, lightweight fabric, such as brushed cotton for cold weather, cotton sheeting for hotter weather, or muslin. Take care not to overwrap your baby as this will increase the risk of Sudden Infant Death Syndrome. A minimum of four will be necessary. These can easily be made by the novice sewer, by hemming a 90 cm x 100 cm (36" x 40") piece of fabric. Cotton sheeting usually comes in wider widths.

The most practical **bibs** are made of towelling and are long enough to cover most of your baby's chest. The number needed will vary, depending on whether your baby vomits frequently. Remove any plastic backing that is not bonded to the towelling, as it is a suffocation hazard to your baby. Do not leave the bib on the baby when putting him down to sleep.

Multiple births

If you are expecting more than one baby, you will have to be very organised before your babies arrive. When you are organising equipment, try to borrow as much as possible. The Multiple Birth Association in your state will hire out equipment and give you practical advice. If you are expecting twins, you will need one and a half times the quantity of nappies and clothes recommended for one baby.

PREPARING FOR YOUR BABY

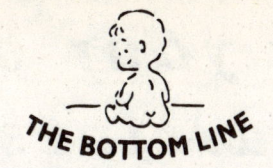

THE BOTTOM LINE

- Inform yourselves about pregnancy, birth options, baby and child care.
- Arrange physical and emotional support for yourselves for the early weeks after the birth of your baby.
- Don't buy lots of very small garments; newborns can grow out of them within a ridiculously short time.
- Learn resuscitation and first aid skills and have a first aid kit prepared.
- Childproof your house.

CHAPTER 2

After your baby arrives

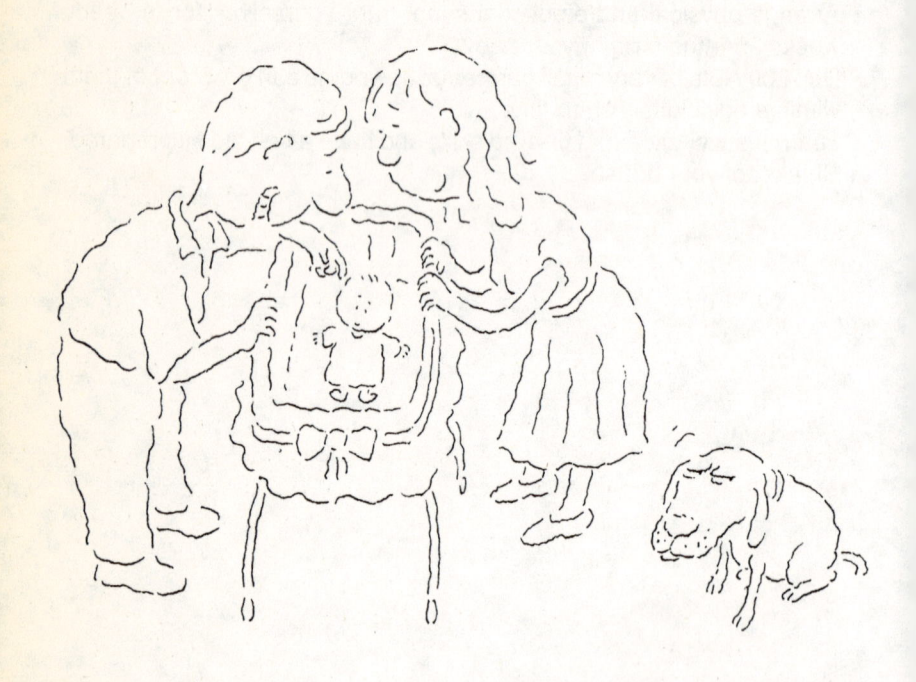

Having a new small life in your hands will be both a rewarding and a life-changing experience. If you have read the 'Preparing for your baby' chapter you will have some of the basic equipment on hand, and, we hope, some useful contact numbers and some idea of where to find helpful people. Even if you are well prepared, you will find that drastic changes, both physical and emotional, occur after the birth of your baby.

This is a time for being very patient with yourself and your partner. Both of you may be new to parenting, and you should not feel embarrassed about needing assistance and reassurance from each other and from outside sources.

Advice

One of the complaints we hear most frequently from new parents who come to Tresillian is about the amount of conflicting advice and information they receive from friends, relatives, health professionals, the media and even well-meaning people in supermarket queues.

Much of this advice can be perfectly practical and well-founded; there are many ways to care for babies and small children, and most parents have their own favoured methods. Some of it, however, consists of little more than myth or superstition. Often, too, it is quite simply unwelcome; new parents trying to establish a routine of caring that suits themselves and their baby can find themselves confused and upset by constant 'helpful' comments.

If you start to get confused, pick one person in whose knowledge and skills you have confidence, and stick to his or her advice. You are certainly under no obligation to try every baby-care method suggested to you, although in the early days it can sometimes be worthwhile to try a few different ways of organising yourself to see what suits you best. Don't chop and change to such an extent that it upsets you or your baby; if something works for you, stick to it.

In many situations you will already have the answers to your problems in mind, but will just need to discuss your solution to check it out. Always trust your own instincts to be right. After all, parents are the people who know their baby best, and after a while will develop a reliable idea of how she will respond in most situations.

When you are consulting health professionals for advice, it is easy to be sidetracked and to forget to ask the questions that were really worrying you, especially if you are holding a restless or crying baby. It's a good idea to write your queries down and take them with you, checking before you leave to make sure you have covered all the points you intended to.

If the information you receive from the nurse or doctor is complicated or you are upset or distracted at the time, it's important that you ask for it to be written down. Then you will have an accurate record of the information you have received and the steps you should take to remedy the situation, so that you can refresh your memory.

Many books have been written on childcare and development. Before buying reference books it is worthwhile borrowing copies from friends or the local library, to check whether the information and advice is suitable for your family. You should also feel comfortable with the tone of the book.

Any advice you receive, no matter what the source, should have the right 'feel' for you. Ask yourself whether the practice being recommended is safe (offering your baby solids before four months, for example, is not a good idea) and whether it is practicable for you (elaborate remedies that require excessive self-sacrifice on the part of the parents should be avoided). Is there an alternative method that is more sensible for you to use?

Remember when you are listening to advice about parenting that every baby and family is unique. Advice that has worked well for a friend's family may not work as well for your family; on the other hand, methods that were useless for a friend may be just what your baby responds to.

Physical changes

For mothers, there are physical changes to cope with as the body returns to normal after the massive adjustments of pregnancy and birth.

The **uterus** usually returns to its normal size and position over about six weeks. After about ten to fourteen days it can no longer be felt above the pelvis.

One of the important signs that the uterus is returning to normal is the **lochia**, or post-delivery discharge of blood. The discharge goes through three stages:

- a heavy red discharge, usually lasting four days;
- a watery pink discharge, usually lasting a further four days;
- a yellowish-white discharge, usually lasting a further two weeks.

The amount of the discharge is determined by several factors, including the size of the placental site (if you have had twins there may be a heavier discharge) and the presence of retained membranes and parts of the placenta in the uterus—these will affect the ability of the uterus to contract. Breastfeeding also stimulates the uterus to contract, and the discharge of lochia may increase while the baby is at the breast.

If the discharge remains red after five days, increases suddenly, is offensive or is accompanied by pain or discomfort, immediately seek the advice of your doctor or midwife. Occasional spotting of bright blood can occur after increased or strenuous activity; this is an indication that your workload and activity level should be decreased. Do not hesitate to seek the advice of your doctor or midwife if you have any concerns about the discharge.

Be prepared for the discharge of lochia with several packs of super-sized sanitary pads. The use of tampons is not advised until after the post-natal medical check six weeks after delivery, as there is a risk of infection arising from their use.

After-pains are due to the contraction of the uterus after the delivery of your baby. These contractions are nature's way of preventing uncontrolled bleeding, as they close off the blood vessels. They usually occur during the first seven to ten days after delivery. The degree of pain experienced is different for each woman, but can be more severe after second and subsequent babies. The pain can also be more severe during breastfeeding or handling of the baby; the release of oxytocin at these times stimulates the uterus to contract.

To manage the pain at feeding time, try doing relaxation exercises prior to and during the feed (see page 57) and take a mild pain-relieving tablet such as paracetamol to lessen the discomfort. Take no more than four doses of the recommended quantity in twenty-four hours, or as recommended by your doctor.

Other pain

An **episiotomy** is a surgical incision in the perineum, the area of skin between the vagina and the anus. An episiotomy is usually performed to allow easier delivery of the baby, to prevent an uncontrolled tear of the perineum or to protect the delicate head of a pre-term infant or the head of a breech delivery baby. Stitches may be necessary after either an episiotomy or a perineal tear, and these require the same kind of care as does any surgical wound.

The midwife will recommend regular salt baths or the use of a hand-held shower, to cleanse the perineum several times during the day. The use of a hairdryer on a low setting to dry the perineum after washing is also recommended, but take care not to burn yourself. This will assist in preventing infection, as well as giving some relief from pain.

It is important to be as comfortable as possible. In hospital, an air cushion should be requested; at home, use an air cushion (these can be hired from the chemist) or a soft pillow to sit on. Use of a mild medication for pain relief, such as paracetamol, is perfectly all right; small amounts of medication will be present in your breastmilk.

Constipation can become a problem. If you have discomfort moving your bowels, increase your intake of fruits and fluids, especially dried fruits; prunes are an excellent bowel stimulant, but take care if you are breastfeeding, as they can make the baby's bowel motions loose.

It takes a while to recover from a **caesarean section**. In the first few days you will be uncomfortable and find normal movements restricted by pain. It may help to apply gentle pressure over the wound with your hand when you move, cough or laugh. If an unexpected caesarean section was necessary, both of you may have feelings of anger, failure or disappointment, especially if you had set great store by having a natural birth. Such feelings are only to be expected, but as long as both mother and baby are going to be well in the long term, you should both try not to let your disappointment cloud your appreciation of your new baby. Discuss any negative feelings you have with someone you can trust. Do not be too hard on yourself, and accept any help that is offered. When you go home with your new baby, take care not to lift anything heavy.

Backache is a common problem for parents, particularly mothers. The physical work of parenting should not be underestimated. Lifting heavy baskets of washing, manipulating prams or strollers up and down stairs, walking the floor with a distressed infant for several hours or just regularly bending over to change your baby's nappy or pick her up, all place strains on your back that may never have been encountered before.

It's important when buying your nursery equipment to check that you will not have to stoop when attending to the baby. This is a problem with most prams, especially if you are tall. You should not have to lean forward to push a stroller or pram. If you have a low change table, invest in a stool to sit on while changing your baby. Make a conscious effort to bend at the knees when picking things up off the floor, lifting your baby or doing household chores. Practise good posture, sitting straight in chairs and walking tall.

Post-natal exercises

Many women are disappointed after their babies are born, having imagined that they would return to their normal shape and weight within days, if not hours, of the delivery. Sorry, this does not usually happen! A regular exercise programme and a well-balanced diet are necessary for the recovery process.

Post-natal exercises should be commenced as soon as possible after your baby has been born (see pages 40–2). The doctor should be consulted first if you have had a caesarean section or a difficult delivery. The midwife or the hospital physiotherapist will be able to suggest suitable exercises if you are unsure how to begin.

One of the most important exercises is that for the pelvic floor muscles. These muscles are responsible for supporting the uterus and bladder; if they are not strengthened by exercise after delivery, complications of incontinence (leaking of urine) or prolapse (dropping) of the uterus can occur later in life.

Six-week check

Most doctors and midwives like to see you for a check-up six weeks after delivery, to make sure that your body is returning to normal. Sometimes your baby will be checked as well. Tell your doctor or midwife if you have any worries at this time.

Parental sleeping problems

The frustration of not being able to go to sleep in the initial days after your baby has arrived is not uncommon. Many women experience an inability to sleep in the first few days—it may be due to the excitement of becoming a parent, combined with all the physical changes that are occurring. If you are in hospital, you will be trying to sleep in strange, often noisy surroundings, and probably missing your partner.

Try to rest as much as possible during the day. Have a warm drink of milk just before bedtime, and a warm shower or bath. Listening to a relaxation tape may help. Avoid drinking alcohol, coffee or drinks containing caffeine. If you continue to have sleep problems, it is important that you speak to your doctor or early childhood health nurse, as you may be developing post-natal depression (see chapter 5).

Your partner or a supportive friend may be able to help you get some sleep by taking care of your baby for several hours during the day. You will probably sleep more soundly if he or she takes the baby on an outing during those hours. Try to take cat naps at other times. An excellent use of occasional care centres is to leave your baby and go home to enjoy a couple of hours of uninterrupted sleep. At first you may find this quite difficult to do, or feel guilty about doing it, but reassure yourself that you need your sleep if you are to cope with your new baby.

Occasionally, even when you lie down and the conditions are ideal for taking a nap, you may not be able to sleep. Console yourself that you are at least resting with your feet up.

If your sleep deprivation is due to your baby being unsettled, seek assistance before you reach the end of your tether. Start with the services offered locally, such as your early childhood health nurse or your local doctor. They will offer advice and support, and can refer you to other sources of assistance if necessary.

Partners may also have sleeping difficulties, especially if you are

POST-NATAL EXERCISES

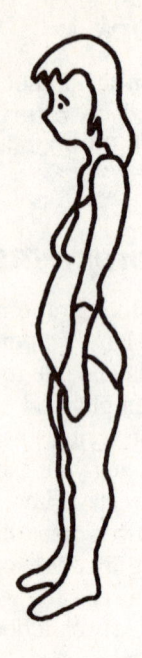

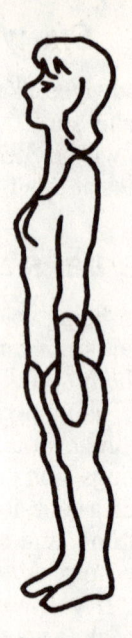

Good posture

1. Posture
Good posture means standing with your **feet** parallel to each other, your **pelvis** tucked up and your **pelvic floor** firm, your **stomach** pulled in and your head up.

2. Pelvic floor exercise
This exercise should be continued for the remainder of your life, to ensure strong pelvic floor muscles.
(a) Tighten your buttock muscles; hold your thighs together.
(b) Draw up your pelvic floor muscles, as you would if you needed to pass urine but could not find a toilet.
(c) Count to five slowly, then relax the pelvic floor muscles.
(d) Repeat five or six times.
Do this exercise several times a day, as often as you think of it. You can get into the habit of doing it at specific times, such as when you are washing up or whenever you go to the toilet.

Exercises 3 to 7 should be done lying on the floor or bed with your **knees bent**:

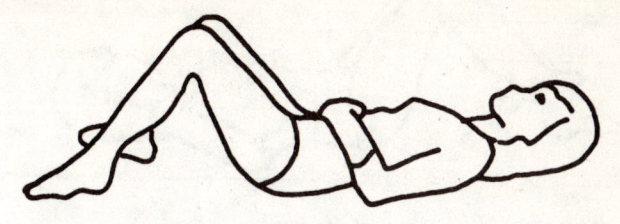

3. Abdominal muscles
Breathe in, allowing your abdomen to rise, then breathe out, pulling in the muscles of the abdominal wall firmly. Then relax.

4. Progression for abdominal muscles
(a) Tighten your abdominal muscles and raise your head and shoulders off the floor, then touch your knees with your fingers. Hold while you count to five, then relax.
(b) Tighten your abdominal muscles, lift your head and shoulders and reach down with your right hand to touch your right ankle. Repeat, touching your left ankle with your left hand.

5. Diagonal abdominal muscles
Tighten your abdominal muscles, then lift your head and shoulders off the floor and reach with your left hand across to the outside of your right knee. Repeat, touching your left knee with your right hand.

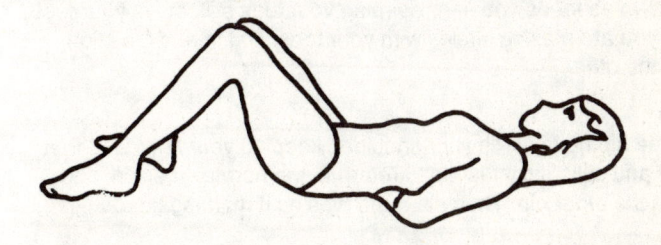

6. Posture control
Place one hand in the small of your back and tighten your buttocks and abdominal muscles as you flatten your back. Hold this position, then relax.

YOU

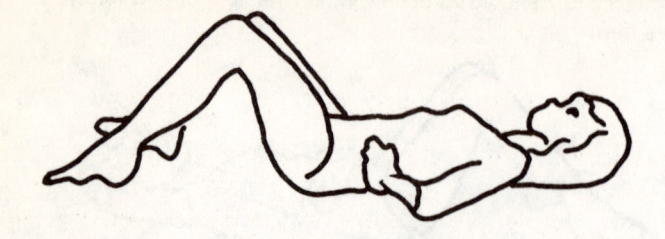

7. Combination abdominal/pelvic floor exercise
Draw up your pelvic floor, tighten your buttocks and pull your stomach in tightly, flattening the hollow in the small of your back. Hold, then relax. Tighten the pelvic floor muscles, place your hands on your sides at the waistline and blow out hard, making a hissing noise.

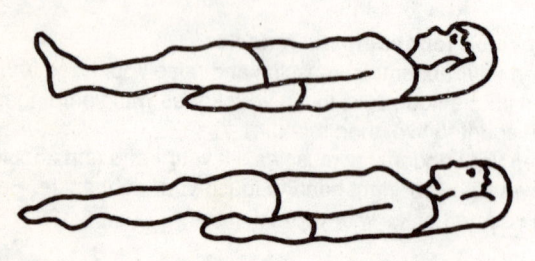

Your knees should be straight while doing the following two exercises:

8. Feet
Bend your ankles so that your toes point up at the ceiling, then point them down as far as you can. Keeping your legs still, move your feet so that you are making circles with your toes, first in one direction, then in the other.

9. Hips
Hitch one hip up towards your shoulder, keeping your knee and foot straight and still. Allow the hip to return to the normal position, and hitch up the other hip. Then alternate hips as if marking time.

Do these exercises once a day for at least six weeks after the birth of your baby. You should also spend some time every day lying on your stomach with a pillow under your pelvis, to aid circulation and to help your uterus return to its normal size.

Adapted from post natal exercises recommended by King George V Hospital, Sydney.

sharing the care of the baby, or your baby needs attention frequently during the night.

Resuming sexual intercourse

There is no fixed rule as to how soon after the delivery of your baby you can resume an active sexual relationship. Factors that will influence your decision will probably be mostly related to the new mother's physical state. If an episiotomy or a caesarean section has been performed, the wound may be painful for some time after delivery. If there is heavy post-delivery bleeding or discharge, neither of you may feel inclined to have intercourse. If either of you are feeling anxious or tired, which is almost inevitable soon after becoming parents, this may deplete your sexual energies. If your contraceptive method is not adequate, worries about a second pregnancy may also inhibit you both.

It is important that you allow yourselves time to physically and emotionally recover from the delivery of your baby before resuming sex, and only you can decide what is an appropriate time. Any period of abstinence is a time when physical closeness of other kinds will be very important to you both, and in the weeks following the birth of your baby reassuring hugs will be beneficial for both of you. If one of you is not ready to have intercourse, there are many other ways to stimulate and satisfy one another. When you do resume intercourse, start off gently and be prepared to notice some differences in sensation until your body has returned to normal.

Sheer exhaustion on the part of one or the other partner is likely to interfere with his or her enjoyment of intercourse; afternoon naps may be necessary to solve this problem. Vaginal dryness is common for many women during the first eight to ten weeks after delivery; this may be compensated for by the use of a lubricating cream available from your chemist. Leaking breastmilk during intercourse is common for breastfeeding mothers, and can be due to pressure on the breasts or a let-down of milk accompanying sexual excitement. Be prepared with a towel to protect the bed.

You may find yourselves being constantly disturbed by your baby when you attempt intercourse, which can be very frustrating and make you reluctant to persist. If this is a problem, make a note of when the baby has a longer, more settled sleep period and use that time to be together. It may be at a time you are unaccustomed to, such as in the morning or the early evening, but, as flexibility and innovation are excellent qualities for the new parent to develop, don't let this chance go by!

You may feel that some of the spontaneity of your relationship has been lost if you need to allocate a time to be together in this way. Be assured that you will regain it as your baby grows and develops a more normal routine, and your energies and confidence return.

One or both of you may simply be uninterested in resuming a sexual relationship after the baby is born. A new father may be nervous about hurting his partner, and both parents may simply be too tired to want to bother. It is important to seek professional advice if one or both of you continue to avoid intercourse for much longer than is necessary and normal for you, as this can be a sign of stress or post-natal depression and can put your relationship at risk. Your early childhood health nurse can refer you to your local family planning clinic, a social worker or a doctor to whom you can talk about your feelings.

Being parents demands that you continually cater to the emotional and physical needs of your baby. It is important that partners also fulfil some of each other's needs to be nurtured and loved. If you are living alone, or your partner is frequently absent, and you are feeling lonely and isolated, you will need to set aside time to devote purely to yourself and your own needs. If you are missing physical contact, a regular massage can help, and your early childhood health nurse will be able to direct you to a professional counsellor for emotional support.

Contraception

It is possible to become pregnant again quite soon after delivery, even if you are breastfeeding. Leaving it until the six-week post-natal check-up to discuss your contraception needs may mean leaving it too late. The method of contraception you use is up to you and your partner; the most commonly used methods are discussed below. Abstinence from sexual intercourse is still the only 100-per-cent safe way of avoiding falling pregnant, as no other method is free from potential failure through human error. If you feel unable to talk to your doctor about contraception, contact your local family planning clinic for information and advice.

The most effective methods are the contraceptive pill or mini-pill, condoms, the diaphragm or the intra-uterine device (IUD).

There are two types of **contraceptive pill**, taken by the woman. The combined pill contains two hormones, progestogen and oestrogen, which stop the release of an egg from the ovaries each month. It is usually taken if you are bottlefeeding your baby. The mini-pill or progestogen-only pill is the one to take if you are breastfeeding. It works by changing the composition of the mucus at the entrance of the uterus, stopping the entry of sperm. It is important to take the mini-pill at the same time each day to maintain its effectiveness. If any side-effects become apparent, seek advice from your doctor or local family planning clinic. Some babies react to a change in the taste of breastmilk when their mothers start taking the mini-pill by refusing the breast for several days or not gaining weight for the first week after commencement.

A **condom** works by collecting sperm, preventing it entering the uterus. The condom is a thin latex sheath that is stretched over an erect penis. It is an effective barrier method of contraception, as long as the condom is in good condition (not perished) and care is taken when putting it on and taking it off. Protection can be increased if spermicidal creams are also used by the woman. Condoms have the added advantage of protecting against sexually transmitted diseases, including the HIV (AIDS) virus.

A **diaphragm** is a soft rubber cap that is worn inside the vagina and fits over the cervix. The diaphragm must be left in place for eight hours after intercourse. A family planning nurse or your doctor will fit you with the diaphragm and teach you how to use it. If you used a diaphragm before your pregnancy, you will need to be refitted, as your cervix usually changes shape and size after pregnancy. Diaphragms are usually not recommended for use for six weeks after delivery, so an alternative contraceptive method should be used during that time.

An **intra-uterine device** is a small plastic or plastic-and-copper device inserted into the uterus. It works by irritating the lining of the uterus, which prevents the implantation of any fertilised egg. The IUD can cause heavier menstrual bleeding, abdominal cramps or discomfort, and there is a risk of uterine infection involved in its use. If you are considering using this method, make sure you use some other method until the IUD has been inserted, which is usually not until at least six weeks after delivery.

Apart from these four methods, there are a number of less effective methods of avoiding pregnancy. There are various **natural family planning methods**, including the Billings, mucus, temperature and ovulation methods. These may not be reliable until your hormonal balance has returned to normal, and they require both partners' co-operation if they are to work. Your local Natural Family Planning Association, family planning clinic or doctor can help you obtain the counselling and education necessary to use these methods successfully.

Spermicidal creams, gels, foams or vaginal tablets can be placed in the woman's vagina prior to intercourse, but they are not reliable as a form of contraception.

The **withdrawal method's** success is dependent on the man withdrawing his penis from the woman's vagina before he ejaculates. This requires a degree of control and an effort of will on his part, and consequently there is a high risk attached to the method as a form of contraception.

Fully breastfeeding, that is, not offering any other fluids or foods to your baby except breastmilk, is sometimes used as a form of contraception. This method works on the principle of maintaining high hormonal levels in the body. Problems can and do easily occur with this method. Feeding must take place at frequent, regular intervals, and life is not perfectly regulated with a small baby. We would not recommend this method of contraception.

The **morning-after pill** should only be used in an emergency, if you think your usual method of contraception has failed, or you have not used contraception and think you may become pregnant. If ovulation and fertilisation have occurred, the pill changes the hormonal balance of the uterus so that implantation cannot occur. If ovulation has not occurred, the pill slows down the process so that the sperm and ovum do not meet. You should visit your doctor or family planning clinic to obtain the pill within three days after intercourse, sooner if possible, if the pill is to be effective.

Sterilisation is a permanent method of contraception. There is no guarantee that the operation can be reversed if you change your mind. In women, the fallopian tubes that connect the ovary to the uterus are cut and tied (this is called 'tubal ligation') so that the eggs cannot come into contact with sperm. In men, the tube that leads from the testes is cut and tied, preventing the sperm reaching the penis (this is termed 'vasectomy'). This does not prevent ejaculation during intercourse.

Maintaining your relationship

Of course, sexual intercourse is only one part of an adult relationship. You may well find that, due to the baby's constant interruptions or your own exhaustion, the usual lines of communication between you and your partner break down to some extent, or seem to carry only messages about the baby's welfare and the methods you are using to care for her. These messages are undoubtedly important; they are a vital part of your adjusting to your transformation from being a couple to being a family. But unless you can perfect the art of conversing in short snatches, you should set aside time each day to talk to each other about each other's personal needs and concerns. While the baby is feeding quietly is a good time, or while you are out walking; try to choose a time when neither of you is too tired to think clearly or to be sympathetic or affectionate.

It is particularly easy for a new mother to become totally absorbed with the care of the baby, and in fact she may be under pressure from all and sundry to do so. This can make even the most devoted partner feel resentful and excluded, and it is very easy for that resentment to be translated into anger towards both mother and baby. If this is happening, it is important that you both spend a little time together away from your baby, and that your partner discusses these feelings with a counsellor if they remain unresolved.

If friends, neighbours or family have offered to babysit, take them up on their offers, and make the effort to have a night out together if you can. If that seems like an impossible feat, given your low energy levels, organise a takeaway meal so that the time one of you would have spent cooking can be spent together. A picnic in a local park may be enough of a change in routine. Take advantage of an occasional care centre to free you for a couple of hours from the distractions your baby presents. Don't be too ambitious in trying to resume your pre-birth social life, but don't stop socialising altogether. Staying at home all the time with only the baby and each other for company is not recommended.

One thing you will probably want to discuss is the birth of your baby. Coming to terms with this special and unique event is a large part of adjusting to being a parent, and your feelings about it will probably carry over into your early attitudes to parenting. For many parents, the feelings about the birth are joyful and celebratory, but for many others uncertainty or dissatisfaction about how the birth was handled by doctors or midwives, or how they themselves behaved, can predominate. It is important that this is voiced and dealt with as early as possible.

If your birthing experience did not fulfil your expectations or plans, talk together about your perceptions of the experience. If this does not resolve your worries or feelings of dissatisfaction, seek professional assistance from your midwife, early childhood health nurse or doctor.

New parents' groups can be a great source of support. If you went to antenatal classes, you and your classmates' mutual curiosity about your babies may draw you together to form an informal post-natal group after your reunion. Talking to these new parents can be very reassuring as you may find that they suffer the same uncertainties and frustrations, as well as the joys, that you do. New fathers may find support and assistance with their feelings in talking to each other or to other support people; watching a woman you love suffering pain can be a disturbing experience, which you may need help to recover from.

Bonding

A great deal has been written about bonding lately, and the result can be that new parents feel like failures if they do not experience a great gush of maternal or paternal love the moment they set eyes on their baby. The fact is that, as with any important relationship, getting to know your baby will take time.

You have had nine months to develop your relationship, but the dreams you have had of your baby may not quite match the reality. Often the baby may have features you did not include when you imagined her, such as funny ears or a nose that reminds you of someone you don't particularly like. This is quite normal. It's important not to be too hard on yourself or feel guilty for being disappointed about your baby's appearance. Spending time with and caring for your baby will help you both to get to know one another. If you are the parent of twins, don't think that it's uncommon initially not to relate equally to both babies. Different temperaments, and even the fact that one baby may be healthier than the other one can make a difference.

Bonding can be assisted by feeding your baby in the labour ward and, if possible, avoiding being separated from her in the early days. Lots of contact with her will help you gain confidence in handling her. Lots of hugs certainly never go astray! If you are having feelings that are overwhelming you, especially feelings of despair or anger, talk to someone about these feelings.

Emotions can be confusing things for new parents. As a mother you may feel excited, happy, tearful, anxious, fearful or overwhelmed, all in one day. As a partner this may be upsetting, as you can also be overwhelmed by all the changes, expected and unexpected, that are occurring. The changing emotions you are both experiencing are normal for new parents, no matter how well prepared you may be for parenthood.

The most important thing to do is give yourselves time; don't make heavy demands on yourself or each other at this time, and try to maintain a sense of humour. Read chapter 3 on survival techniques, and use some of the suggestions there to help you cope. If you continue to feel out of control of yourself or your situation, it's vital that you ask for help, either from a friend or relative you know you can trust or from your early childhood health nurse or other professionals with counselling expertise.

Premature babies

Often, the parents of a premature infant have mixed feelings about the birth of their baby, ranging from joy at her arrival to guilt that they have in some way caused their baby to be born early. Premature infants look different from full-term babies, and it may take a little while to get used to the fact that your baby is small, fairly thin, perhaps not as well as you would have hoped, and not much like the baby you had imagined you would have.

Try to visit your baby frequently while she is in the hospital; it is important that you get to know her as closely as possible by sight and, if possible, by touch. Ask the nurse to take a photograph of your baby so that you can show the photo to your family and friends and look at it yourself when you are away from her. Leave a picture of your family with your baby so that you can feel you are there with her in some way, even when you have to be physically absent. Express breastmilk if you can, and take it to the nursery for her. Take your friends and relatives in to visit your baby, so that they too can begin to get to know her. Starting a diary and recording all the small developments and changes in your baby's condition can help give you a real sense of her progress. Other parents with premature babies can provide reassurance and practical support.

The special care nursery staff are experienced with small and sick infants and with the anxieties of parents with small babies, and will help you in every way they can, as well as explaining the equipment they are using and their treatment of your baby. Do not hesitate to discuss with them any worries you may have about your baby.

In the first few weeks, depending on her weight, your baby may need to be tube fed, as premature babies often have poor sucking reflexes. These will improve as she gets bigger. Expressed breastmilk can be given to her until she is old enough to feed directly from the breast.

Most premature babies do very well after the initial stages, and grow normally.

Babies with special problems

Nothing can prepare you adequately if your baby has some type of major health problem. As parents you will experience a wide range of emotions, including being overwhelmed by the adjustments that will be necessary to cope with your child's condition, and anger at the destruction of your expectation of bearing a healthy child. These feelings can affect all members of the family, as well as close friends, and, however intense, are normal. You need to discuss them with a social worker or other health professional when you feel able.

There are support services available in the community both for your baby and for yourselves. At first, you may not wish to discuss your baby's condition or even to acknowledge her birth, but it is important to remember that you are not alone.

Try to get as much information as possible about your baby's condition, and do not make any decisions until you understand this information and are in control of your feelings.

Partners should try to be supportive of each other and discuss their feelings with each other if possible. Do not be afraid to ask close friends for help and to accept any reasonable help that is offered.

Separation from your baby

Separation of either parent from the new baby, for whatever reason, can be distressing. If she has been hospitalised, it is important that she has the reassurance of your presence as often and for as long as possible. Discuss the hospital's policy with the staff, and if necessary negotiate prolonged visiting times or overnight stays with your baby. In paediatric wards, nurses will happily accept the presence of parents with their babies. Parents provide comforting, secure arms for upset babies. The accommodation for parents will vary from quarters situated in the hospital grounds to an armchair beside your baby's cot.

If you notice any changes in your baby's condition, tell a nurse. Make sure you voice your concerns to the nurses and doctors and have your questions answered. It is important that any fears you may have be laid to rest as soon as possible so that you can effectively care for your baby. Give yourself a rest every now and again; if you don't want to leave your baby without a familiar face around, arrange with your partner to take it in turns to sit with your child, or have a friend or relative visit, so that you can get some relief from the stress of long hours of waiting and watching.

If your baby is to undergo a painful procedure that you will find difficult to sit through, leave the ward. Be ready to come back and give her lots of cuddles after the procedure is over. Ask to see a social worker if you are finding the hospitalisation of your baby difficult. Social workers are skilled in helping parents communicate their fears, and in arranging emotional, physical and, if necessary, financial support.

Always check with the nurses before giving your baby anything to eat or drink. Remember that you are part of a team of people who are caring for your baby.

A breastfeeding mother can continue breastfeeding during her baby's time in hospital, either directly or by expressing breastmilk to be fed to

AFTER YOUR BABY ARRIVES

the baby by the staff or by her partner or a support person.

Understand that an older baby will be upset when you have to leave and she cannot go with you. You will no doubt be upset yourself, but you should not stop visiting as a tactic for avoiding these painful minutes. It is important for both parents and baby that you visit as regularly as possible. An older baby may be comforted by having an article of clothing that you normally wear, to hold or sleep with.

If you have an older child, be open and honest with him about your baby's condition. If you have to leave him to visit your baby, don't sneak out whatever the hour, kiss him goodbye and say when you will return. He will probably cry, but this is better than him finding you gone without any explanation.

A breastfeeding mother who is hospitalised can continue to breastfeed, by having the baby room in with her, by having the baby brought to visit her for regular feeds, or by expressing breastmilk at regular intervals to be given to the baby (keep a photo of the baby handy to help you express). Check with the doctor that any medication you are taking cannot harm the baby if transmitted through breastmilk. If you are very ill, rooming-in will not be an option open to you, and you may not be able to continue breastfeeding. You should take good care of your breasts, regularly checking them for areas of discomfort while you are weaning. See chapter 12 for more information on weaning.

If you cannot have the baby with you, arrange for her to be brought to see you as often as possible so that you can see that she is safe and well, and hold her if you are well enough. This advice is applicable for hospitalised fathers, too. For the times when separation is unavoidable, have some of your favourite photographs of her to look at .

If your partner needs to spend time away from the family, arrange for a friend, relative or support person to phone or visit you every day. If possible, cook extra servings of casseroles, spaghetti sauces and other meals that freeze well. This will help ensure that you eat well when you are on your own. Arrange occasional care for your baby, if you have not already started to use this excellent service, to give yourself well-deserved time out.

When the family is reunited once more there will be a new set of adjustments to make, so don't expect everything to return to normal straight away. The hospitalised parent or child may still be quite ill, in which case the household will have to be reorganised to make provisions for caring for him or her. Expect a little more stress than usual for everyone involved, and accept any useful form of help that is offered by friends, relatives or neighbours.

Your toddler and the new baby

If you have an older child, you will need to continue the work you began while preparing him for the arrival of the new baby, so that problems of resentment and jealousy are minimised.

When you are in hospital with your baby, have your toddler visit you. He will probably be upset that you cannot come home with him, but it is important that he sees that you and the baby are well. Make a fuss of him when he visits and have a small present ready for him. Save the packets of biscuits from your tea tray or have small packets of dried fruit made up in advance, as presents to give your toddler when friends arrive with presents for the baby. Add a balloon to the package, so that he has something left to play with after eating the biscuit or fruit.

When you are leaving the hospital, walk with your toddler, and let your partner or support person carry the new baby.

Once you have arrived home, allow the toddler to hold the baby. Make sure that the baby is secure, but try not to seem too anxious about the toddler's ability to hold her. If he is rough, phrase your corrections in a positive way. 'Pat the baby gently' is more helpful than 'Don't hit the baby!', 'Hold her a bit more tightly' less alarming than 'Careful, you'll drop her!'

Allow your toddler to help you care for the baby, carrying the nappies or getting small articles for you. Try to give him a clear idea of his usefulness and his place in your family. Encourage your visitors to spend some time with him as well as with you and the baby, so that he doesn't feel he's missing out on attention. While the baby is sleeping during the day, try to spend time playing with him, or create time for this by having your partner or someone else mind the baby while you and the toddler go to the park or on some small outing.

When you are feeding the baby, always know where your toddler is; have something for him to do, where you can see him, while you feed.

Don't expect behaviour and understanding that are beyond the toddler's capacity. Remember, toddlers do not understand concepts such as sharing, or the helplessness of a newborn baby. The decision to have a new baby was yours, not your toddler's, and it is only natural that occasionally he will feel that the new situation has been forced upon him, and perhaps suggest that the baby be sent back to where it came from.

Try to be as consistent as possible in your rules. Continue using the same rules and discipline that you used before the new baby arrived. This will help your toddler feel secure in the changed circumstances.

Your pets and the new baby

If you have an animal that has lived with you for some time, it is possible that it will be jealous of the new baby. Approximately half of the dog bites on children are caused by the family dog.

To prevent problems with **dogs**, continue your normal routine, your daily walk or your normal greeting when you arrive home. Introduce your dog to the new baby. Often animals come off second best with small children, but this is not always the case, so keep a close eye on any interaction between dog and baby and be prepared to intervene at a second's notice.

Care should be taken with **cats**, as they can curl up next to your baby in the bassinette and pose a risk of suffocation. Their presence may also aggravate any allergies and respiratory problems your baby has. It is a good idea to make a habit of closing the baby's bedroom door when she is asleep to prevent this happening.

Make sure you wash your hands well after handling animals, before you pick up your baby, and keep your animals healthy with immunisation and regular worming and de-fleaing.

See pages 238–9 for other safety measures to take if you have pets.

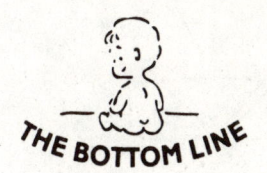

THE BOTTOM LINE

- Take time to care for yourself.
- Cuddle and spend time with your baby.
- Make time to do your post-natal exercises and have your six-week check.
- Use the survival techniques and support services available.
- Talk to your early childhood health nurse or doctor if you are having trouble sleeping, even when your baby is settled.
- Find a regular time to spend with your partner.

CHAPTER 3

Survival techniques for parents

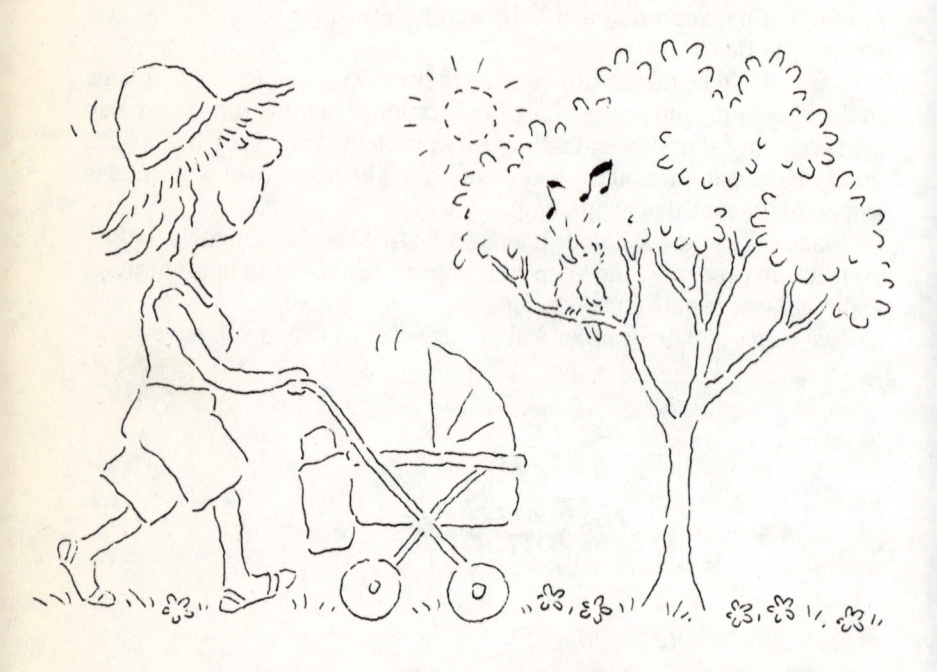

Before we have children ourselves, everyone has ideas about what parenthood involves and what parents are capable of, ideas which have been developing since we were small children. Many such ideas are based on our observations of our own parents, and these observations are supplemented by powerful media images of parenting, as well as our own increasingly mature observations of the way parents behave in the real world.

The main problem with the kinds of happy fantasies that we tend to develop of ourselves as parents is that they are usually not very realistic or practical. Movies, television and all types of advertising project images of parents who are endlessly calm and patient, consistently well-groomed, and who attend to their baby's and their partner's every need. Their houses are always tidy, no matter what the time of day or night, and they always manage to have the time and the energy to build fulfilling careers, to socialise and to enjoy recreational activities of various kinds. These images are not at all realistic, and trying to reproduce them in real life places you under great physical and emotional strain and can result in tension in all your relationships.

The great majority of new parents do a fantastic job. At times you may feel frustrated, confined or just plain unsuited to your new role, and this can be reflected in feelings of anger and confusion towards the baby. But once the first shock of adjustment is over, creating a routine that allows you at least the bare minimum of recreation time will generally lead to the easing of such feelings.

Adoptive parents go through many of the same difficulties as natural parents; even though adoption agencies do what they can, the impact a baby will have on a household is often impossible for the new parents to imagine before his arrival. Like all parents, you will need time to get to know your baby, and you are bound to feel at some stage that being a parent is not as you expected it would be. Don't expect too much of yourself too early, and if you feel overwhelmed or angry with your baby, talk to a supportive person, such as your early childhood health nurse, an experienced telephone counsellor or the staff at your adoption agency.

When things are not going well with you and your baby in the first few months, try not to be totally disheartened. There are many measures you can take to cope. Some involve 'networking', that is, actively maintaining your contact with the outside world; others entail coming to terms, within yourself, with the changed circumstances that parenthood has brought. Let's deal with the latter first.

Maintaining a positive outlook

First of all remember that you are new at this job, and, as with any new job, you have to allow for an extended period in which to develop and fine-tune your skills. Most occupations require you to serve a long apprenticeship or to have years of study and experience behind you before allowing you to assume the full weight of your responsibilities. Parenthood, on the other hand, demands that you act as managing director from day one. While this may be a rare opportunity, it comes at a time when you are physically and mentally perhaps least prepared for such a major challenge!

Give yourself time; don't expect too much of yourself, whatever messages you are receiving from anyone else. It is arguable whether parenting is a job in which you can ever expect to be perfect, but certainly you will reach a stage where you feel more or less comfortable with the idea of being a parent. If you have not yet reached that stage, persistence is the only means of getting there. And along the way, there are rewards you never dreamt of before you became a parent.

When you are finding it difficult to cope, try to take life one day at a time, and don't plan to achieve more than you can handle in that one day. Set small, achievable goals in the early days—these may be as simple as having a bath, doing the washing up, or sitting in the garden for an hour or so—and be prepared to change them if you are simply too tired, or your baby refuses to sleep, or someone visits.

Try to see such changes of plan as proof of you developing the flexibility necessary for being a parent, rather than as failures to fulfil your own expectations.

Try to find something positive, or at least humorous, even in near disasters; almost anything that has unsettled you will look less dreadful when viewed as a learning experience. For example, when your baby continually brings up milk on your freshly-laundered clothes, the advisability of always having a clean cloth covering your shoulder will be brought home to you!

Impossible as it may sometimes seem, enjoying at least some of this time as a new parent is very important. You may be longing for the time when your baby responds to you with actual words and co-ordinated gestures, but keep in mind that there is a lot of joy to be had in caring for a tiny baby, too. Live in the present as much as you can, and try to make the most of it. The developments during the early months, which sometimes can only be distinguished by a baby's parents, pass with lightning speed, even if at times they do seem to be unending.

When things go right, make sure you acknowledge your involvement and achievement. When you have accomplished some small feat during the day, such as getting on top of the washing, or doing the supermarket shopping (with or without the baby), congratulate yourself. Sometimes it helps to do this out loud.

Start each day afresh; things may have gone badly yesterday, but every day is a new one. Tell yourself you are doing a good job. Be confident that you are the best parents your baby could ever have.

If you are feeling angry and frustrated with your baby, tackle your feelings head-on; you can do nothing to change them until you have properly acknowledged them. Pretending that things are going well when you feel you are losing control will only worsen the situation. Sometimes you will only become aware of your feelings in conversation with another person, so it is important to maintain contact with other adults. See the 'Keeping in touch' section, on page 59.

Practical measures

Learn to relax. Relaxation is not simply an attitude of mind; there are specific techniques you can use when you are feeling tense, angry or restless. Simple relaxation exercises need take no more than a few seconds, and can make the difference between losing your temper and remaining reasonably calm and in control of things.

Take care of your own physical needs; eat well and exercise regularly. Get adequate amounts of sleep whenever possible. In the early days this may mean parents sleeping in shifts, or snatching a nap while the baby sleeps during the day. Take the phone off the hook when you are having a daytime sleep, but warn anyone who is likely to call that you will be doing so.

Continue with your post-natal exercises until you are happy that your body is restored to 'normal'. If you are unsure as to how long to continue, make an appointment with your midwife, physiotherapist or doctor. If you are exercising, the process of returning to normal can take anywhere from six weeks to six months. If you are not, it will take much longer and problems are more likely to arise later, especially with regard to your pelvic floor muscles (see page 40 for pelvic floor exercises).

Protect your back. Parents of babies and small children have to do a great deal of bending and heavy lifting, so it's important not to strain your back. Remember always to bend at the knees rather than from the waist when you are lifting anything heavy. New mothers should be particularly careful, and avoid all strenuous lifting.

A QUICK RELAXATION TECHNIQUE

This takes only a minute or two and can save you from hours of stress.
1. Breathe out with a long sigh, dropping your shoulders as you do so.
2. Relax your face, unclenching your jaw. Become aware of your facial muscles, eyes and forehead, and try to relax them.
3. Keep your breathing easy and quiet.
4. Repeat this technique again, and as often as you feel is necessary.

Use a nappy service, or disposable nappies, for at least the first month to give you some extra time. If neither is within your own budget, suggest to relatives or friends that they might like to provide one or the other as a combined present.

Establish priorities for housework and baby care. What housework do you think is absolutely essential? If you must have a made bed or the washing up done, attend to that first when you have the time, for your own peace of mind, but leave other chores for later. Partners can make a joint list and share the chores, if they don't do so already. If you are alone, make sure that only what is absolutely necessary for your own and your baby's health and hygiene is included on your housework list for the early weeks of parenthood. Washing nappies, making sure that you always have clean dishes, and keeping yourself and your baby clean are probably the most essential tasks. And accept that if you are enjoying playing with your baby, this activity is more important than the housework. Don't waste time feeling guilty about all the tasks that await your attention.

Parents of twins or triplets should put housework at the bottom of their list of priorities and take care to have the nursery set up so that everything is on hand.

Try to keep the lounge room clean and tidy, even if this means that you just put all the mess in another room for the moment. This will help you feel more organised when visitors call. Most people who venture further than the lounge room will be friends who should understand the chaos that accompanies the arrival of a new baby.

Most visitors will want to help you in some way, but will not want to intrude. Write a list of things that need to be done around the house and put it on the fridge, so that if anyone offers help you will know immediately where to direct their efforts. Folding nappies is a great job for visitors.

Let visitors get their own tea and coffee, and have a good supply of packet biscuits on hand for them.

Try to tidy as you go, putting things back where they belong as soon as you have finished with them rather than leaving them out to be tidied up later. If this is not practical, put things that are waiting to be tidied away into a neat pile or a large basket, and cover with a sheet or towel to give a superficial impression of tidiness. Don't dry the washing up; cover it with a teatowel and let it drip dry.

Wear clothes that need little ironing and do not crush easily. After washing and drying, either fold them and put them away immediately or use them straight from the washing basket. Leave the ironing that you

SURVIVAL TECHNIQUES FOR PARENTS

will not need immediately, until you or your partner have spare time to deal with it. If your partner does not already help with the domestic chores, he will become better at it with a little practice—try not to be too critical of the initial results.

Be efficient with your own energy when cooking. Make and freeze casseroles, meatloaves and other foods that only require reheating. Foods such as chicken, cold meats, cheese, tomatoes, yoghurt, baked beans, peanut butter sandwiches and fruit, especially apples are easy to prepare and nutritious. A boiled egg with toast and a drink is filling, nutritious and quick to make. Tinned fruit, meats and vegetables can save you time, too. Set aside one night a week for takeaway food and have your partner or a friend pick it up on the way home from work.

If your budget will allow it, consider a live-in mothercraft nurse, nanny or housekeeper for the first seven weeks. If this is not possible, try to make arrangements for friends, relatives or neighbours to help you with the housework, or to mind your baby while you shop.

Allocate time each day for resting, and playing with and enjoying your baby. Occasionally declare an entire day housework-free and spend it indulging yourself and your baby.

Try to go out at least every two days, even if it's only for a walk around the block. If it's raining and miserable, ring up a friend for a chat, just to take you mentally out of the house for a while. Even a ten-minute call will make you feel fresher and less isolated.

It's important that you get some time to yourself. There may be an occasional care centre in your area that has trained staff to look after your baby for short periods while you shop or do the housework or catch up on a bit of sleep. You should also claim some recreational time for yourself, out of sight and hearing of the baby if possible. Have your partner or a friend take the baby for a walk and have a relaxation bath with all the trimmings, read a book or a magazine or just sit with your feet up enjoying your own uninterrupted thoughts.

Photocopy and fill in the 'Contact Numbers' on page 14, put it by the telephone and use it—don't hesitate to ask for help as soon as you look like needing it. There is specialised help, physical and emotional, available to you, and you should feel free to take advantage of it.

Keeping in touch

For your own sanity, try to make contact with at least one other adult every day, either by phone or in person. You may have an informal chat with a neighbour as you go to the mailbox, or you may have a standing arrangement with your partner or a supportive friend or relative to talk on the phone at least once every day.

If you live in a caravan, a home unit or a block of flats, introduce yourself to your neighbours and let them know that you have a young baby in the household. This personal touch can prevent problems of neighbour relations if your baby is particularly unsettled—most people will refrain from complaining about being disturbed by a baby crying if they know you personally.

To keep things in perspective, try to go out with your partner or a close friend for at least one hour each week, leaving your baby in the care of a relative, friend or babysitter. Take coins or a phone card for the telephone the first few times you do this, because you will probably want to ring to check that the baby is all right.

If you are in a relationship, take time to be together and devote time to voicing your own needs and listening to one another's physical, practical and emotional needs. Going out together to dinner or lunch can help you focus on your life as a couple independent of your baby, and need not always exclude him; a picnic in the park or a snack in a coffee shop while he sleeps in his pram can provide enough of a break in your routine. A walk around the block together will amuse your baby and give you time to talk. If you find it absolutely impossible to talk freely when the baby is present, set aside some time for talking when he is asleep, or arrange for someone to mind him for a little while.

Make an effort to meet other parents in your community who have babies of a similar age. Join the local parents' group or attend a playgroup (often run by the local early childhood health or community centre) so that you have regular contact with other parents. Talking with them can reassure you of just how normal you and your baby are, and it can be a relief to confide in others about how difficult it is to be a parent sometimes! You can also pick up some practical tips about various aspects of baby care.

Be friendly and say hello if you meet another parent in the local park. Many people who are isolated feel that they will be a nuisance if they talk to others, but if you are polite and not overbearing your company will be welcome. You can begin by showing an interest in the other parent's baby. If you get along well, and you run into each other again, suggest meeting again, perhaps in the park or at a coffee shop. If your suggestion is refused, try not to be too disheartened to try again.

When cultivating new friendships, be friendly, approachable and a good listener, but remember that you need to share some of yourself, and that you are entitled to have your say as well.

STAYING SANE

Take a large sheet of paper and make a list of things that make you feel contented, less stressed, more relaxed and happy, that help you to cope and feel good about yourself and life.

Don't be too selective at first; put down anything that comes into your head, from 'travelling' to 'eating out' to 'soaking in a long, hot bath'. Put down activities that are now pretty well impossible with a baby, like 'browsing in the shops' or 'inviting all our friends around for dinner'.

Now go through the list and try to think of ways of adapting all of those activities to your new circumstances. Travelling any great distance might be impossible, but a day's outing with the baby and a picnic lunch to a national park or local river might provide the stimulation of new surroundings and a break from the house. Cooking a big meal for all your friends might be impossible, but having a couple of people around for a light supper—particularly if they bring the food!—can help you keep in touch with the outside world. 'Sleeping all day' could become a two-hour afternoon sleep while the baby is in occasional care.

Try to indulge in at least one of the activities on your list every week.

If you live in a remote area, have your support network set up in case of emergency or for times when parenting is difficult. Try to use the resources in your area, such as the early childhood health nurse and the local hospital and community staff. Arrange to meet other parents with new babies in your region. This may involve travelling long distances but will be worth it.

It is tempting to compare your baby with other babies, especially if they are similar in age, and to measure his progress against theirs. To some degree this is harmless, but it can be destructive, especially if parents are out to impress. It simply does not matter that someone else's baby smiles three weeks before yours does, or that yours utters his first word two months before theirs. As long as your child is happy and appears to be encountering no serious difficulties in mastering the basic skills, you should not worry.

There are probably older people in your community who would be delighted to be visited. You can find them through community centres, senior citizens' centres, church groups and voluntary agencies.

Local community or church groups often set up activities during the day that you may like to attend, such as painting, pottery and craft classes. They often have cheap or free babysitting services, or there may be occasional childcare in your area that you can use to enable you to attend. If you have a hobby or a special interest, join a local group or class; this is a good way to meet people. Now that you have a baby you will have to be organised in advance to attend meetings, but you will probably find that it is worthwhile to have a regular break from babyminding.

Talk about your feelings to a sympathetic listener, especially if you are worried or have feelings of losing control. The staff of Parent Help Lines are aware of the stresses facing new parents, and are equipped to help you with understanding and advice. Most parents will confess to having felt like this at some time during their early experiences of parenting. If these feelings continue or become all-consuming, it is important that you seek advice from your doctor or early childhood nurse. You may be suffering from post-natal depression. See chapter 5, 'Post-natal depression', if you think this may be so.

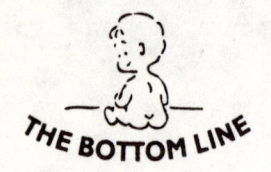

THE BOTTOM LINE

- If you need help, it is available and you should use it; remember, you are not alone in your parenting.
- Major changes in your life always require a lot of adjustment. Be kind to yourselves and don't expect to always get things right first time.
- Perfection is impossible: 'good enough' will just have to be good enough during the early weeks.
- Think positive, be practical and stay in touch with the outside world.
- Try to retain your sense of humour.

CHAPTER 4

Coping with crying and lack of sleep

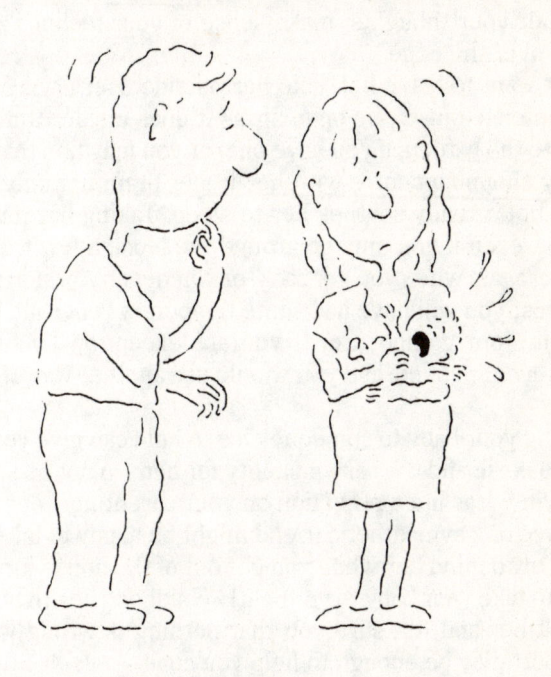

There is probably nothing quite so upsetting to new parents as the sound of their own baby's crying. Onlookers will not be anywhere near as disturbed as you are, and may even be able to muster sympathetic smiles or offer to hold her for you if you are clearly in difficulties. So try not to become distressed about her disturbing others, on top of worrying about what is causing her to cry.

Similarly, neighbours may not even notice your baby's crying, unless she is very persistent. If you live in a confined area such as a flat, home unit or caravan, let your immediate neighbours know that you have a new baby and to apologise in advance for your baby disturbing them. Most people will be sympathetic and patient if approached personally.

If you cannot establish what the problem is (a later section of this chapter, 'What to do if your baby won't settle', provides an exhaustive list of possibilities) and your baby will not stop crying, do something before you get to the stage of smacking or shaking her. Go somewhere where you cannot hear her crying for a few minutes; put her in a safe place and take a short walk outside, or have a shower, wearing a shower cap and allowing the water to fall on the cap to drown out the crying. A few minutes without the sound of her crying may be enough of a break for you to gather your thoughts, make sense of your feelings and stop yourself going over the edge.

If you don't want to leave her, take her outside. Her crying will not sound half as intense out in the open air as it does inside. You can just take her out into the garden, if you have one, or you may find that a stroll through a busy shopping centre with her in her pram not only drowns out the crying but actually soothes her to sleep. Taking her for a drive may soothe her, even if you only go around the block a few times. She may start crying again when you get back, or whenever you stop at traffic lights, but at least you will have had some temporary relief and this will help you regain your composure. If you are exceptionally tired this method is not recommended, and you should use another way of settling your baby.

Simply giving your baby to someone else to hold can give you a spell of rest from the noise and the responsibility for her. Do not be surprised if she stops crying. It is not a reflection on your parenting. Your partner, a visiting relative or a sympathetic friend might be happy to take her for a walk for you, or to mind her while you get out of the house for a while. You may want to take your baby to your early childhood health nurse and have her check her and reassure you that nothing is wrong with her; often this support may be enough to help you cope.

If it is the middle of the night, there are 24-hour Parent Help Lines available, and you should not hesitate to use them if you are having problems or feeling unable to handle things.

Remember, before she learns to speak, crying is your baby's only method of communication. Babies cry for some reason, even if it is only boredom. Try hard to remember that your baby is not doing this deliberately to upset you, even though it may feel that way.

Your baby's sleep

Many baby books will tell you that babies sleep twenty hours every day. Let's set the record straight—they don't! If you, like most parents, take about an hour to change, feed and settle your baby, assuming that everything goes well, and that you feed about six times a day, this leaves only eighteen hours in each day for your baby to sleep. Subtract the two to four hours during which your baby will probably be unsettled, which is fairly average, and you only have between fourteen and sixteen hours left for sleeping on a good day.

Each baby is different, and some need more sleep than others. The amount of sleep your baby has is not a concern if your baby settles well and has regular periods of sound sleep. If your baby sleeps longer than sixteen hours each day, be thankful for your good luck!

Most new parents are painfully aware of the sleeping patterns of their babies, because in the early months these patterns totally disrupt their own sleep. The good news is that 70 per cent of babies develop reasonable sleeping patterns by about seven weeks of age and will by then 'sleep through the night', which really means settling at about 11.00-11.30 at night and expecting a feed at about 4.00-4.30 in the morning. You will be surprised at how grateful you will be for this meagre amount of continuous sleep.

What to do if your baby won't settle

The idea that babies eat and sleep continuously is a myth—if it were true, they would not be able to walk, talk and be as sociable as they are by twelve months. *It is normal for most new babies to have a period of two to four hours daily during which they are unsettled, and at least one unsettled day a week.* These periods ensure that they get attention and stimulation, which helps them grow. It has nothing to do with your parenting skills, whether this is your first or fourth baby, whether the pregnancy was planned, whether you wanted a girl and got a boy or vice versa: it is normal behaviour for all babies. The only problem is that the timing of the unsettled periods does nothing for your sanity; you will probably find that you do not care very much about your baby's social skills as you vainly try to settle her at 3.30 a.m.

Your baby will sleep better when she is loved, fed, warm and dry. It is not possible to spoil a baby under twelve months of age by picking her up or giving her cuddles.

Your baby may protest for a short while before going to sleep, for no particular reason. This is quite normal. If your baby has taken a good feed and is still unsettled, you need to consider other reasons for her not sleeping. She may have problems with **wind**, or be **cold, hot, wet or bored**.

Most small babies, if bottle fed, need to be 'winded' or burped. You might try burping your baby halfway through a feed as well as after the feed. The most efficient method is to hold your baby on your lap, making sure that her back is very straight. Rest a hand on her tummy and hold her gently. It is not necessary to pat or rub her back to bring up the wind, but you may feel comfortable doing so. Just before the wind comes up your baby will usually wriggle; do not change her position at this stage. It is sometimes worth waiting for a second burp.

If you have held your baby in this position with no success for five minutes, resume the feed or, if the feed is finished, put your baby to bed, or give her a cuddle. If you are breastfeeding you may find that your baby will pass wind through her bowel. This is quite normal.

Raising the head of your baby's bed slightly when she sleeps often helps to settle her, as most babies experience a small amount of **overflow of milk** from the stomach into the oesophagus when they are small. This can be done using a small pillow *under* the mattress.

Sometimes your baby will be **thirsty** because she has been crying, because the weather is hot or because she is overwrapped. You can give her cooled boiled water at this time. The water should be boiled for five minutes and then left to cool. Give about 60 mL (2 fl oz) in a bottle with a slow teat. If you prefer, there are special water teats, slower than other teats, which are available from chemists. The water needs to be at room temperature or just above. Check to make sure that it is not too hot (it should feel lukewarm on the skin on the inside of your wrist) and that the teat is not too fast (the water should drip through the teat at a rate of one drip per second). Discard any water left in the bottle that your baby does not drink.

It is handy to keep a supply of cooled boiled water in the fridge for these occasions rather than waiting for the water to cool while the baby is unsettled, especially if you live in a hot region. Discard any leftover boiled water after twenty-four hours and prepare a fresh batch, to reduce the risk of bacteria multiplying in the water.

Most babies sleep and settle better if they are loosely **wrapped**; wrapping helps your baby feel secure. Take care not to overwrap because of the risk of Sudden Infant Death Syndrome. She has come from a very confined and warm environment in the womb, and the open spaces of the outside world can be unsettling for her. This is one reason why your baby will probably sleep better in a bassinette. If it is extremely hot weather, wrap her in a light cotton or muslin bassinette sheet rather than a bunny rug or cuddly. When wrapping your baby, allow room for her arms to be flexed.

Remember to lay her down on a different side after each feed.

In the summer months you can dress your baby in just a singlet and a nappy to sleep. Babies lose their body heat easily when they are small, and especially if they are premature, so a singlet is essential even in very hot weather. In the winter months the use of a bonnet and bootees, and sometimes mittens in very cold weather, will help your baby sleep. A sleeping bag is useful for older babies, who tend to wriggle out of their blankets.

Clothing that has lace, frills and buttons may look cute when your baby is out visiting, but it is not always the most comfortable to sleep in, just as sleeping in your best dress or a three-piece suit is not comfortable for you. All-in-one baby suits and soft nighties are better for small babies, as they are stretchy and comfortable, and will also cut down on the ironing you need to do. Natural fibres such as cotton are best. Cellular cotton blankets can be used in the bassinette as they are light and warm and can be tucked in firmly to help your baby feel secure.

To counteract boredom don't leave your baby wrapped up all the time. Give her lots of **floor exercise** every day. This helps to strengthen the muscles of her neck, shoulders and arms, and enhances her development. Lay her on her tummy with her arms outstretched beside her head, so that she can lift her head. Place a toy or something interesting for her to look at 20–30 cm (8–12") from her face, and do not leave her for too long in the same position or she will become bored. You can get down on the floor yourself and play with her at this time. If your baby is very new, several minutes at a time is probably long enough. Putting her in the washing basket with a folded up blanket on the bottom will be a change for her, and the basket will be easy for you to move from room to room with you.

Small babies should be placed in a different **sleeping position** each time you put them down, so that their heads develop evenly. Place your baby on either side, but not on her front as research has linked this practice with cot death.

The room can be **warmed** with a heater if the weather is very cold. Hot water bottles can be used to warm the bedding, but should *not* be used when the baby is in the bassinette. Electric blankets should never be used for small children, because of the risk of burns, overheating, dehydration and electrocution.

A fan can be used to cool your baby's room in extremely hot weather, but should not blow directly onto the baby. Overhead fans are of more use if you live in a very humid region, as they circulate the air well. If you use a floor fan, make sure that the fan cannot tangle in the bedclothes.

Extreme care should be taken using electrical equipment around small children.

To **keep your baby dry** at night you can use nappy liners, either disposable or reusable (even disposable nappy liners can be washed and reused a few times), or pilchers, preferably without plastic lining. Fluffy cotton-based pilchers, as well as those made of doctors' flannel, are also available. These products will become wet overnight, but they keep the urine from sitting against the baby's skin. When your baby gets older, you may have to use two nappies doubled up to keep her dry at night.

Your baby should be changed at each feed or when very unsettled. Most babies are not disturbed by a wet nappy, but others seem sensitive. A thin layer of vaseline or barrier cream (such as zinc and castor oil) can often help to keep the urine from the skin of a sensitive baby.

If your baby has **nappy rash**, it should be treated immediately. Look for obvious causes, such as the use of plastic pilchers or a reaction to the laundry detergent you are using. Bleaching nappies, and the use of conditioners in the final rinse, can often cause rashes. Thrush, a type of fungal infection, can also cause rashes, and should be treated by the doctor. See page 214 for a description of the symptoms.

The use of a **dummy** can sometimes help to pacify your baby, but make sure that it is not torn or perished and that it is washed and sterilised frequently. It is not advisable to put glycerine, honey or any other sweet substance on your baby's dummy, as once she starts growing teeth the constant contact with these sugary substances can lead to dental caries. It is often helpful to have two or three dummies, so that you can give a clean one to your baby while washing and sterilising the others. Do not attach the dummy to your baby's clothing while at home, as the string or ribbon you use may choke her.

If the crying continues, and you have checked all the above possibilities as causes of her distress, consider the possibility that she is **bored**. Babies, like adults, need stimulation and changes of environment. Moving your baby from one room to another, or placing a mobile over the bassinette for her to look at, can help. Of course, it is also possible that your baby has been overstimulated, and needs to have some of the external stimuli removed.

Colic

The debate still rages as to whether colic exists and, if it does, what causes it. Some experts blame parents' emotional problems and poor feeding techniques. Other theories put forward allergy or food intolerance as possible causes. The baby's temperament also has been blamed. Whether or not colic exists, and whatever its cause, you may find that your baby has a crying period during the day that someone calls colic.

Bouts of crying between six and ten o'clock in the evening may start at about three to four weeks. Your baby turns red, draws up her legs and screams, and no amount of feeding, walking, talking or contact will stop the crying. It stops as quickly as it starts as the baby falls exhausted; about twenty minutes later she wakes to start again. These bouts may go on for hours at a time. This type of behaviour is common in small babies. It occurs in both breastfed and bottlefed babies, and usually lessens by three months of age.

Regardless of the cause, this is a difficult time for all concerned, and you will need to use your survival techniques and try to maintain your sense of humour. You should have your baby checked by a doctor to ensure that there is not some medical problem causing her crying.

It is possible to get medications for treating colic. There are varying opinions about the use and value of such medications. If you feel that medication is necessary, be sure to follow the directions given by the doctor or the chemist carefully, so as not to overdose your baby. Some medications work by reducing the surface tension of the wind in the bowel and relaxing the smooth muscle of the digestive tract so that there are fewer spasms. Some of these also contain alcohol. A prescription is needed from the doctor for some of these preparations. Tresillian does not recommend herbal medicines as some contain sedatives and many have a variety of herbs (the amounts of which are not well regulated), weeds and seeds.

All the methods of settling suggested earlier in this chapter are recommended for babies with colic.

Settling your baby

Your baby may settle if you **sit her outside** for a few minutes with her nappy off. Be careful not to sit her in direct sunlight or in the wind.

Some **gentle music or a relaxation tape** can help to settle her. A relaxation bath may also help. Make the water very deep and make sure the room is warm.

Sometimes a **monotonous sound**, such as the noise the vacuum cleaner makes, can help a baby go to sleep. Vacuuming can also give you an opportunity to tune out for a few minutes if all else has failed. Having done the vacuuming makes you feel in control of the housework, too!

If your baby wants to be near you but you simply must get a few things done around the house, a carry pouch will free your hands so that you can wash up or hang out the washing while your baby feels warm and secure. If your baby falls asleep in the pouch, in her safety capsule or in your arms, put her in her bassinette, even if you are concerned that the movement will disturb her. Capsules and pouches are fairly cramped, and when your baby wakes she will not be as refreshed as if she had slept in her own bed, just as you do not sleep as well on the lounge as you do in your bed.

If you have been pacing the floor with your baby, as new parents are prone to doing, or you have been out frequently and your baby has been having disrupted sleep, sometimes putting her back into the bassinette and wrapping her can help her settle. If she is crying, do not leave her unattended for more than three to five minutes. Sometimes your baby will settle in this time—if she is still awake but quiet, leave her for a few more minutes, as she is quite likely to drop off to sleep.

You can also gently **rock or pat or stroke** your baby while she is settling—a rocking chair is ideal for settling her prior to putting her to bed. It is easy enough to rock her if you have a movable bassinette, but keep in mind that if she gets into the habit of being rocked to sleep it may be difficult to continue once she graduates to a cot. Make sure that your patting is gentle; if you are becoming agitated with your baby's crying it may be safer for you to leave the room for a minute or two. If your baby is still crying and unsettled after three to five minutes, pick her up again and give her a cuddle, and maybe try a **massage**, a **deep relaxation bath** or some **relaxation exercises** (see pages 72–3). The directions given below are suggestions only. Do not be too concerned about following them to the letter; the idea is to help you and your baby relax. You may feel a bit clumsy to begin with, but your confidence will grow as you get used to handling your baby. See pages 72–3 for guidance.

Massage

Massage is one method you can use to settle your baby. Some babies enjoy this more than others, and you may need to introduce it gradually. It is normal for your baby to cry at the beginning of a massage, but most babies will settle after a short time.

You may wish to give your baby an all-over massage or just a limited one around the stomach region. If massage is done to the stomach, it should be done softly, in a clockwise direction and not directly after a feed.

Massage should be done with a small amount of warm oil, in a warm room. Almond, wheatgerm, jojoba, olive or apricot oil, or any other oil that is not highly perfumed, are suitable for use in baby massage. Commercial baby oils usually contain mineral oils, which can be drying to your baby's skin. You will also need two towels, and perhaps some soft music playing to produce a relaxed atmosphere.

Choose a place that is warm and quiet and where you will be comfortable and not likely to be disturbed; take the phone off the hook if you are alone in the house. The floor, a bench over which you do not have to bend too far, or your lap are all suitable places on which to massage your baby. Use the towels to keep the oil from your bunny rug, carpet or lap.

Make sure the oil is warm before you apply it to your baby's skin. You can place it in a small, clean container in another container of warm water. Your hands should be warm too. If they are cold, put them under warm water for a few seconds to warm them. Place the oil where you can easily reach it, but out of reach of any toddlers.

If you live in a very hot region, you will have to apply oil sparingly when you massage your baby, as the application of oil to her skin can affect her capacity to sweat, which is a very important part of the self-cooling process for small babies.

- Remove your baby's clothing and speak soothingly to her. Commence by gently massaging your baby's head with your dry hands.
- Using a little warmed oil, place one hand around your baby's wrist and with the other hand gently stroke her arm from shoulder to hand a few times. Repeat this stroking on the other arm.
- Massage her body from shoulders to hips, using long strokes and making sure that your hands remain well oiled.
- Massage her tummy gently in a clockwise direction, starting at the umbilicus and moving outward. Continue to talk soothingly to your baby as you progress down her body.
- Massage her legs in the same way as you did her arms, with gentle strokes downwards towards the toes, holding her by each ankle in turn and cupping her feet as you go.
- Turn your baby over onto her tummy and massage her back with long, downward strokes, including her buttocks in these strokes.
- Move your hands gently from the centre of her body out over her

RELAXATION EXERCISES

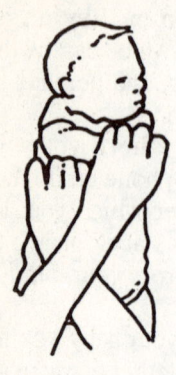

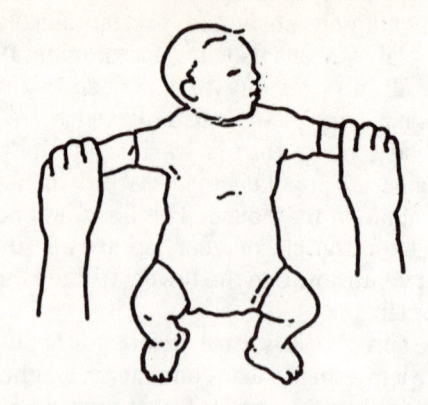

1 Place your baby on her back. Gently hold both her hands and move them into a crossed position over her chest. Then move them out to fully extend her arms, without forcing her if there is any resistance in her arms. Bring her arms back to her chest. Repeat this extending movement five times.

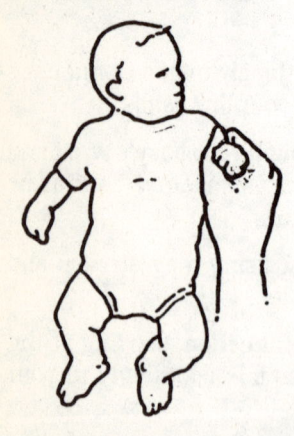

2 Supporting your baby's wrist firmly with your hand, shake her hand gently to relax the grasp. Repeat this movement with the other hand.

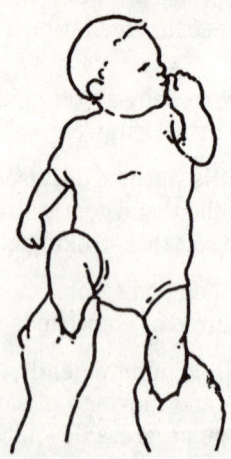

3 Hold your baby's right leg and bend her knee gently towards her tummy. Do the same with the left leg and then gently move both her legs in rhythm, as if she were pedalling a bicycle. Repeat this movement five times.

COPING WITH CRYING AND LACK OF SLEEP

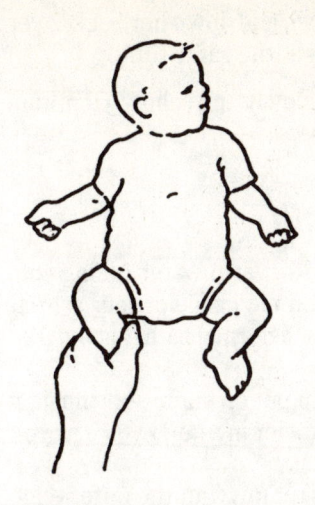

4 Holding your baby's ankle, shake her foot gently to relax it. Repeat this movement with her other foot.

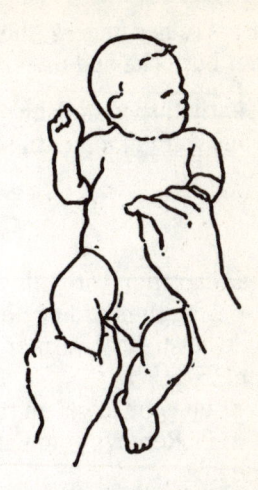

5 Hold your baby's left hand and right foot and gently bring them together diagonally across her body until her hand and her knee touch. Repeat this movement five times. Do the same with her right hand and left leg.

6 Place one of your arms along the side of her body and roll her gently from her back to her tummy and back again, first to the left and then to the right. Repeat this movement five times.

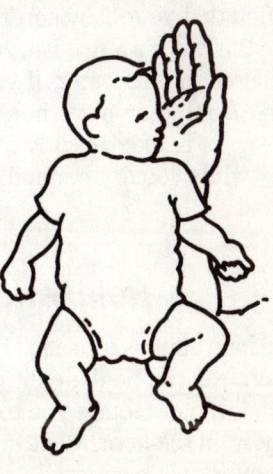

When you have finished, give your baby a cuddle.

arms to her fingers, then back to the centre, and down her back, over her buttocks and then down both her legs at the same time.

- Gently turn your baby over and dress her slowly and calmly. Continue your soft talking until she is fully dressed.

Relaxation bath

For a relaxation bath, fill your baby's bath with warm water (using cold water first, then adding hot). Test the water on the inside of your arm. It should be slightly warmer and deeper than for a normal bath—about 12–14 cm (5–5½").

Set up your towel on the change table and put on some soft music if you wish. Remove your baby's clothes. Talk to her in a quiet voice as you bathe her.

Place your baby gently in the bath on her tummy. Put the outer edge of your hand along her jawline so that your little finger is hooked under her chin, keeping her face out of the water. Her cheek will automatically fit into the palm of your hand and her ear and head will rest comfortably on the inside of your wrist. Spread your fingers slightly apart so that water does not collect against her face, and keep your knuckles clear of the water. Your forearm and wrist should be as relaxed as possible.

Pause and allow your baby to completely relax in the water. You will probably find that your baby settles quickly. You can hold her for several minutes in the water if you wish, unless the bath is distressing her. Never leave her alone in the water. If you find it too difficult to position your baby on her front, then place her on her back. This is just as relaxing.

When she is relaxed, gently lift her from the water, and continue to talk calmly while you dry her and dress her. Be careful that she does not become cold.

Relaxation exercises

Illustrated instructions for relaxation exercises are given on pages 72–3. These exercises can be done either on a change table, if it is a suitable height and does not require you to strain your back bending over, or on a rug or cuddly on the floor. Make sure that the room is warm and that you are in a comfortable position.

Change your baby's nappy so that she is clean and dry to begin with, and make sure that she is wearing loose, comfortable clothing. Remember to talk to her as you do the exercises.

When nothing seems to work

Sometimes you will have exhausted every possibility there is to be checked as a cause of your baby's crying, and cuddled, massaged, exercised and bathed her, and she will still be unsettled. You will probably be tired yourself by this time, and will need to tap into your own resources and use your survival techniques (see chapter 3).

Ring up a friend, relative or one of the Parent Help Lines across Australia or New Zealand to talk to someone who is sympathetic and to whom you can honestly tell your feelings without being judged. If you are alone with a crying baby, put her in another room while you call so that you can hear the person over the phone and respond more calmly.

Parents' groups are a good form of support; sharing your experiences and swapping workable techniques can help everyone concerned.

Be honest with yourself about your feelings. Acknowledge that you are tired, frustrated and angry, and do something safe with your feelings. Putting your baby down in the bassinette, going to your bedroom and pounding a pillow can help get rid of some of your stored-up frustration. When you are all pounded out, take a deep breath and consciously try to relax your body before going back to your baby. (For a quick relaxation exercise, see page 57.)

Parental sleep deprivation

Losing sleep is probably the greatest source of stress for new parents; it is important to recognise this and have some idea ahead of time of what you will do when the sleep deprivation looks like getting the better of you.

If you are in a relationship, it is a matter for discussion whether you are going to allow your baby's night-time feeding or wakefulness to disturb both partners' rest. Keep in mind that if the same partner is always having to get up at night, he or she can build up a very natural resentment at the other partner's always being allowed to sleep properly. The other partner could perhaps return the favour by caring for the baby early in the mornings, or during the night-worker's weekend sleep-ins or afternoon naps.

In the first six to seven weeks, try to get some rest while your baby is sleeping. Take the phone off the hook and have a sleep if possible—if you can't sleep during the day, just lie down and relax or read a book or magazine. You will be tempted to try and get control of the housework, but in these early weeks your being rested is more important than a tidy house for everyone's sanity.

Most importantly of all, be sure to recognise when you have not had sufficient sleep to cope with daily life. If there is absolutely no way you can get the sleep you need, be very, very easy on yourself, your baby and everyone around you. Forget the million-and-one things you feel you ought to be doing: for example, if you have run out of nappies because you are so far behind with the washing, use disposables for the day. If you feel that your partner is not doing enough to help you, try to stay calm while you ask for assistance. If visitors are overloading you with unwanted advice, try to accept it graciously; remember, you are under no obligation to follow it!

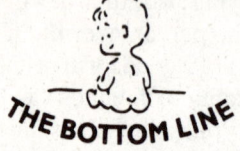

THE BOTTOM LINE

- Your baby's crying is her only way of communicating. Try not to take it as a personal attack on you.
- Check through the reasons she may be crying. If none applies, use techniques that will help you relax as well as soothing her.
- Ask for help; you are not alone. There are services and listening ears available. Early childhood health nurses, and staff on the 24-hour Parent Help Lines of residential hospitals, are aware of the pressures on parents and can give you practical and emotional support.
- In the early months, try to sleep when your baby sleeps. Learn to recognise when you need more sleep and always give sleeping higher priority than housework.
- Don't expect perfection from yourself or your baby: 'near enough' is good enough.

Your Baby

CHAPTER 5

Post-natal depression

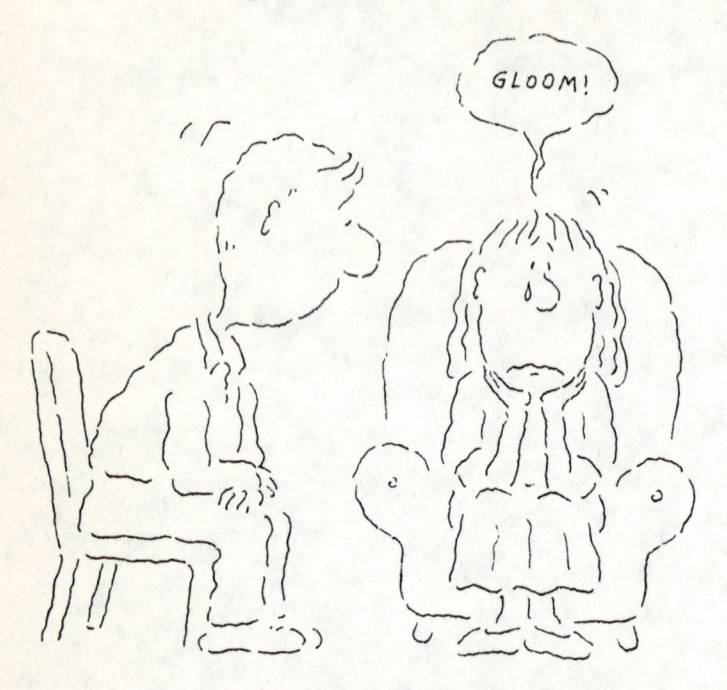

In our society, a woman is expected to function in many roles—as partner, mother, housekeeper, cook, cleaner and nurse, and often as breadwinner, too. The degree of support and assistance you receive from your family, friends and the community may vary from a great deal to very little.

Your worst enemy may be yourself, if you have high expectations of yourself as a mother and are not used to asking for help. There are many unrealistic myths about motherhood and stereotypes of mothers, which all put unnecessary pressure on you. Some of the myths include the following:

- Motherhood is a woman's ultimate fulfilment.
- A mother immediately and automatically feels love for her baby.

- A baby will suffer long-term emotional damage if there is not an immediate bond between mother and baby.
- Motherhood is a time of sublime contentment.
- Women instinctively know how to mother.
- Parenting means mothering.
- Mothers are carers; fathers are providers.
- Motherhood is romantic.
- A mother is selfish if she expresses her own needs.
- Mothers should not go out to work until their children are five years old, because young children need their mother's care.

These myths should be ignored. Being a parent is a lifelong learning process that is different for every family.

Baby blues

Many women are confused by their feelings when they become parents. Your mood may change rapidly from joy and amazement to being overwhelmed by the responsibility of having a child to look after, and tiredness caused by the constant demands of your family.

These feelings are normal in the early days of parenthood — 50 to 70 per cent of new mothers experience mood swings. It is believed that these are associated with the rapid drop in hormonal levels in the body after the birth.

The emotional low points are generally known as the 'baby blues', and should not be confused with post-natal depression. If you give yourself time to physically and emotionally recover after the birth of your baby, these feelings will become more easily controlled.

Symptoms of post-natal depression

During pregnancy and the first year of being a mother, there are many emotional, physical and social changes occurring in your life. These, like all changes, can make you vulnerable to depression.

Health professionals tend to see post-natal depression as a complex condition. Factors that may influence it include the high expectation that women will cope as mothers as well as in the work force, the inadequacy of social supports, obstetric problems or difficulties, marital problems or a mother's poor relationship with her parents. Women are affected regardless of age, class or culture. It is estimated that at least 10 per cent of women in Australia suffer from post-natal depression during the first year of their baby's life.

There are many symptoms of post-natal depression, and they vary from woman to woman. They occur in different combinations and in varying degrees of intensity from mild to severe.

Symptoms may include an inability to do household chores, poor appetite and exhaustion; for some women, being agitated, needing to be constantly busy and being overly concerned about the safety of their families may be a problem. Each woman has different coping mechanisms, needs and strengths.

Many women find it difficult to talk about their needs and how they are feeling. The feeling that you are the only one who cannot cope with being a parent, and that you are a failure, is common. It is important to talk about such feelings to a health professional, rather than continually focusing on your baby; his needs are important, but so are yours, and if you are unhappy it may have an effect on him.

How do you know if you have post-natal depression?

There are several ways to find out if you have post-natal depression.

Talk to your early childhood health nurse or to a doctor who will discuss how you are feeling and the anxieties you have about being a mother. She may refer you to a mothercraft hospital that has expertise in assisting mothers and their families in overcoming post-natal depression, or to a psychiatrist. The role of a psychiatrist is to help you manage the changes you are going through; she will reassure you that you are not going mad.

Read pamphlets and magazine articles about women's experiences with post-natal depression. This will give you further insight into how you are feeling, as well as reassuring you that you are not the only person to suffer from these feelings. Many early childhood health nurses will have pamphlets and booklets on post-natal depression, which they can lend to you. This information may also help your partner understand how you are feeling and your need to seek professional assistance.

All parentcraft hospitals offer a telephone counselling service (see pages 241–2 for telephone numbers). Use this service. You can also talk

SYMPTOMS OF POST-NATAL DEPRESSION

The onset of post-natal depression is signalled by a combination of symptoms, which may include several of the following:

- loss of control when usually competent
- a poor self-image
- a poor sense of self-worth
- an inability to do household chores
- being tearful for no apparent reason
- exhaustion and being overly concerned about lack of sleep
- overwhelming feelings of anxiety or depression
- poor concentration
- poor appetite, or overeating
- a loss of interest in sex
- suicidal thoughts, plans or actions
- an inability to think clearly or find the right words
- fear of social contact
- exaggerated fears about the health and safety of self, baby or partner

to an early childhood health nurse or social worker if you need further help establishing whether you have post-natal depression.

Women who have been diagnosed as having post-natal depression are usually relieved that at last there is an explanation for their unusual or uncontrollable feelings, other than insanity. The diagnosis of post-natal depression is the first step to regaining control of your life. No matter how great the degree of post-natal depression you are suffering, accepting that you need assistance, and sharing how you are feeling, are the first stages in the healing process. The best gift you can give yourself, your baby and your family is to care for yourself.

Partners are usually relieved also, and start to regain confidence in their supporting roles. Couples can start to talk to one another truthfully about their feelings and the special needs they have as individuals and parents.

Treatment

Women recover from post-natal depression to lead happy and productive lives if they are given adequate treatment, support and time. There are various types of treatment available for post-natal depression. The treatment that is best suited to you should be recommended by a counsellor or doctor who has discussed with you how you are feeling and behaving. In many cases a combination of treatments and interventions is needed and recommended.

Individual counselling can be given by a psychiatrist or social worker. In many cases these health professionals work together to help you work through your feelings and anxieties.

Medication is often suggested, and you have the choice of accepting or declining this form of treatment. Anti-depressants are usually the drug chosen. It will take between one and two weeks for this medication to begin to take effect; it needs to build up in your system before the full benefit can be felt. It is important that you take it exactly as prescribed by your doctor. If you experience any unpleasant feelings or side effects while on the medication, contact your doctor for advice. During the first two weeks of taking the medication, you may experience feelings of extreme tiredness. It is important to allow yourself extra time each day to rest, and to ask for assistance with household chores and caring for your baby. If you are breastfeeding, it is important to let your doctor know and to discuss this with him or her as it a factor to be considered when prescribing medication.

The main advantage of **group programmes** is that they make women aware that they are not the only ones suffering from post-natal depression. Other positive effects are that they help women become aware of the amount of community support available, encouraging them to utilise childminding, sporting and educational facilities, and playgroups. There are two types of group programmes: treatment programmes and support programmes.

Treatment programmes are run by skilled group leaders, who help establish the group and maintain its focus or purpose, which is usually the development of skills to better manage depression. These groups have a definite starting date and run for a specified period of time. A commitment is also made by the members to continue attending the group until its completion. Once a programme has commenced, no other women are admitted to the group. The nurses and social workers at Tresillian have been running treatment groups for several years, with a great deal of well-documented success. These groups are now offered in many communities.

Support programmes have no definite starting or finishing date, and there is usually little restriction on group attendance. The focus of the group is usually less clearly defined than in the treatment programme, but women can join or leave at any time. These groups are often very successful at helping women to network in their communities, at building up friendships and counteracting isolation.

Partners

Post-natal depression can cause concern, confusion and anger in a normally happy household. One major problem for the partner of a woman suffering from post-natal depression is the lack of communication that cuts him off from her. You may be quite happy to share the many tasks of parenting, but your partner will not or cannot tell you what type of help she needs or wants with the baby and the house. She may seem very angry but be unable to let you know why.

The anger that is being expressed by your partner may be the result of factors such as frustration with her inability to meet her own expectations of herself as the ideal mother and partner, grief at the death or absence of a close family member, particularly her mother, or anger at the type of delivery she had. At times her anger may leave you feeling confused, upset, inadequate and depressed yourself.

It is important that you help and support your partner throughout the course of the various types of treatment she may require. Discuss with her how best you can help her with the baby and household chores. Make sure that your partner has time to herself and gets adequate amounts of rest. Spend time together as a couple, and show her that you love and appreciate her.

If you are unsure how to help her, or remain confused about what is happening to her, make an appointment to see the health professional who is caring for her. Many men have found that participating in a group for partners is useful, as it helps to demystify some of the feelings they have been experiencing. The sharing of techniques for managing during this sensitive time in your lives may stimulate new ideas or reinforce your confidence that you are doing a good job.

Caring for your baby

Small children and babies can react to the anxieties and moods of their parents. If your baby is unsettled or you are not feeling confident about providing the day-to-day care necessary for your children, seek assistance from your early childhood health nurse. She may refer you to a family day-stay unit or a residential parentcraft hospital.

Accepting help with your baby and/or small children can be a positive step towards regaining control in your life.

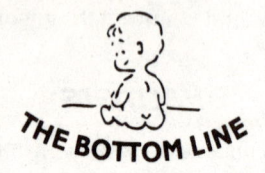

THE BOTTOM LINE

- Try to have realistic expectations of yourself, your partner and your baby.
- Talk to your early childhood health nurse, who will direct you to the appropriate health professionals if you are in need of treatment.
- See page 241 for a list of professional resource centres for post-natal depression.
- Allow yourself time to recover physically and emotionally from your labour and delivery.
- Care for yourself, with time out, adequate nutrition and sleep, for your own and your family's sake. Use your survival techniques when necessary.
- Involve your partner in how you are feeling; suggest that he read pamphlets and magazine articles on post-natal depression.
- Avoid renovating or moving house in the last months of your pregnancy or during the first six months after the birth of your baby, as this will only place additional strain on your family.

CHAPTER 6

From birth to three months

But it doesn't look like the one in the ads!

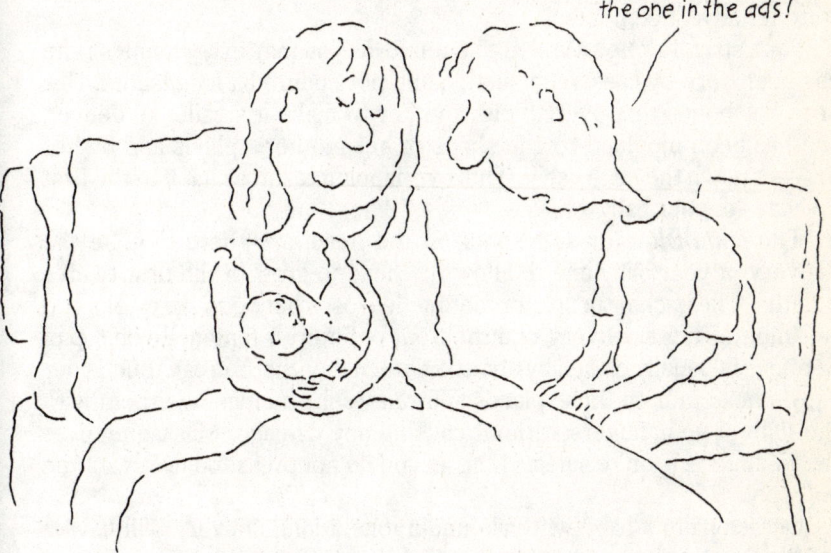

Newborn development
Vision — to about 20–30 cm (8–12")
Hearing — normal at birth
Taste — within a few days of birth
Smiles — between four and six weeks
Responds to mother's voice after first few days

Average sleep
10–16 hours a day
70% of babies sleep through the night (from about 11.30 p.m. to about 4.30 a.m.) by seven weeks

Feeding
Breastmilk or formula, on demand (every 2½–5 hours)

Weight gains
Regains birthweight by 10–14 days
Average 150–200 g (5–7 oz) per week

Immunisation
First Triple Antigen, oral Sabin and Hib — at two months

Your baby's appearance

Your own baby may be the first newborn you have ever seen up close. You may have prepared yourself for her appearance by looking at pictures of newborn babies in books about birth and babies, or you may have been quite happy just imagining how perfect and beautiful she was going to be on arrival. When she does arrive, you may be quite surprised if you expected a baby such as those you admire in baby-powder and fabric-softener advertisements.

For a start, her **head** will not be round, as you may expect, unless she has been born by caesarean section and not endured a long labour. Her head has bones that overlap one another to make it smaller to deliver, and has been moulded by the shape of her mother's pelvis and by her descent down the birth canal. This overlapping resolves itself in the first few days of your baby's life.

The *fontanelles*, or soft spots on the head, are there to ease the delivery of your baby and to allow the head to grow in the first twelve months. The back or posterior fontanelle closes between six weeks and two months after delivery, and the front or anterior fontanelle on top of her head is usually closed by about eighteen months. You can touch your baby's head in both these places and can wash and massage them with the flats of your fingers without causing any damage. Massaging over the fontanelle is quite safe as long as you do not press too firmly on the soft spot.

Occasionally a baby who has undergone a long delivery will have a *swelling* on the back of her head, and this swelling can be very soft and movable. It will go down in the first few days and will cause no problems.

A *cephalhaematoma* is a collection of blood under the bones of the head, and looks like a large bump on one or both sides of the head. It occurs in some babies, and disappears without treatment in about six weeks.

When your baby is first born, her **skin** may look pinkish, bluish or even purplish in colour; any of the three is quite normal. When she breathes for the first time she may become pink and blotchy—her colour will gradually improve until she is a healthy pink within minutes of being born. Take care to keep her warm, as newborn babies have problems initially with regulating their temperatures.

Milia are pinprick-sized white spots that commonly occur over the nose and other places on a new baby's face. They are caused by a blockage of the glands that oil her skin. They disappear within the first few weeks and need no treatment.

FROM BIRTH TO THREE MONTHS

Birthmarks are caused by a collection of blood vessels close to the surface of the skin. As babies' skins are fairly transparent at birth, birthmarks are easily seen on the surface of the skin. The most common birthmarks are referred to as *stork-marks*, a reference to the myth that babies are delivered by the stork. These are usually found on the back of the neck, on the eyelids and occasionally on the forehead. They usually fade by the age of two years and require no treatment.

Mongolian spots are a bluish-black colour, not unlike a bruise. They are mostly on the lower area of the back and buttocks, but occasionally can be in splashes over other areas of the skin. They are common in babies whose parents have darker skins, and will fade by about two years.

Another common type of birthmark is the *strawberry mark*. This starts as a flat, red area in the first few weeks after birth, but then grows to resemble a strawberry in size, texture and colour. Strawberry marks are usually harmless, and will slowly disappear, leaving a small red area. They should be examined by a doctor to ensure that they are not attached to an internal organ. Once this is done, no other treatment is necessary.

Any other birthmarks should be examined by a doctor.

In some babies, the **tongue** is attached to the bottom of the mouth at birth by a fine piece of skin—a condition commonly called 'tongue tie'. This usually causes no problems, as the skin grows longer as your baby gets older, and does not usually require surgery.

When your baby is newborn, the **genital area** may be swollen. This is normal, and the swelling will go down in the first week. Occasionally baby girls have some menstral spotting, which is not a cause for alarm.

Slight turns in newborn babies' **feet** are common, and result from the position of the baby in the womb. They are particularly common in breech births. Most don't require treatment, but they should be looked at initially by the doctor to make sure that the bone structures are normal. Some foot exercises are sometimes necessary, but if the turn is severe it may require surgery.

Umbilical cord care

Treatment of your baby's umbilical cord varies depending on where you live. In some areas minimal cord care is advised while in others surgical methylated spirits is used—be guided by the advice of staff at your hospital. The umbilical cord will take approximately one to two weeks to separate from the umbilicus. If using surgical methylated spirits, the cord should be treated at every nappy change. The methylated spirits should be put at the base of the cord with a cotton tip, but you should avoid putting it on the surrounding area as it will irritate your baby's skin. Some parents find this task a little off-putting, but the more frequently the cord is treated, the earlier it will fall off. Wash your hands before attending the cord. The nappy should not cover the umbilical area; this helps keep the area dry and helps the cord come off earlier. If minimal care is advised in your region, then dry the cord with a cotton tip after your baby's daily bath. If the cord becomes sticky or smelly, commence using surgical methylated spirits.

It is not uncommon for there to be a small amount of spotting of blood when the cord separates. If there is more than a few spots, apply a cottonwool ball with some methylated spirits to the navel and have the area checked by your doctor or early childhood health nurse — otherwise, discard the cord. Any redness or swelling should also be checked by the doctor.

Umbilical hernias (weaknesses in the abdominal muscle wall) sometimes occur in small babies and they are common in premature infants. These do not normally need any treatment, and most have disappeared by the age of two years because of the strengthening of the abdominal muscle as your baby becomes more mobile. It is not advisable to place strapping or coins on the hernia, as these do not help the muscle to strengthen and only make the baby's skin red and sore.

Tests performed on newborn babies

A score out of ten (her **Apgar score**) is given to your baby shortly after she is born. The midwife attending will note your baby's colour, her heart rate, her muscle tone, her breathing and her cry, at one minute and again at five minutes. The Apgar score gives any medical professional dealing with your baby an idea of her condition at birth, and can be useful for reference if health problems occur in the future.

It is essential that a newborn screening test called a **Guthrie test** is performed on your baby to detect the presence of any rare metabolic disorders and some inherited diseases. The test is usually done on the fourth or fifth day, and in most states is used to detect the presence of phenylketonuria, galactosaemia, hypothyroidism and cystic fibrosis. The test involves taking a little blood from your baby's heel; the blood is sent to a laboratory for analysis and the results are known within a few weeks. You will only be contacted if there is a problem with the test and the laboratory needs to repeat the test. Often this is because insufficient blood was collected for the first test, or the test paper was contaminated in some way. Most results are normal.

Phenylketonuria is a rare condition that, if untreated, causes developmental delay. It is an inherited condition in which the protein in both breastmilk and formula milks causes damage to the baby's brain. A special formula is needed if babies with phenylketonuria are to grow and develop normally.

Galactosaemia is a rare condition in which there is an excess of galactose, a milk sugar, in the blood. This condition is treated with a special formula free of galactose, and babies with this condition grow normally.

Hypothyroidism is a rare condition in which the thyroid gland is absent, small or not functioning adequately. Treatment is commenced early with a thyroid hormone and the baby grows normally both physically and mentally.

Cystic fibrosis is a condition that is common in Caucasians. It is caused by a faulty gene and is inherited from both parents. Children with cystic fibrosis have a problem with salt imbalance. They have abnormal mucus production, which affects their lungs, causing breathing difficulties, and also problems with the absorption of food, and causes bowel problems. Children with cystic fibrosis have recurrent infections. Early diagnosis and treatment help reduce complications.

When your baby is first born, her liver is immature and the level of red blood cells in her body is very high. These red blood cells break down within the first few days of her life, and the liver sometimes has a little trouble coping with the breakdown. Your baby's skin can become yellow as a result — this condition is called **jaundice**. Many babies become jaundiced on the second or third day, and this usually takes about a week to clear.

If your baby is jaundiced in hospital, a serum bilirubin test (a blood test for which a small amount of blood is taken from the baby's heel) may be performed to determine whether treatment is required. This will be decided by the doctor. You will be told about this test before it is performed. If the jaundice has not resolved completely after two weeks, another test may have to be performed.

Immunisation

Diphtheria, tetanus, rubella, poliomyelitis, measles, mumps and whooping cough are all serious illnesses. They broke out periodically in epidemic proportions before the introduction of immunisation programmes designed to control them, and there have been outbreaks since, when community levels of immunity were low, leading to the deaths of many children. Within the past few years there have been outbreaks of whooping cough, causing distress for parents and concern for the community at large. Concern over the side-effects of immunisation, and public misinformation and over-emphasis on such side-effects, resulted in the community's level of immunity dropping, causing an outbreak of diseases, especially whooping cough. What is important is that your baby is immunised against this serious condition. It is still possible for your baby to get these diseases, but having her immunised significantly decreases the risk of infection.

Triple Antigen injections are given to your baby at two months, four months, six months, eighteen months and prior to entering school (between 4 and 5 years of age). These injections protect her against diphtheria, tetanus and whooping cough, and the **oral Sabin** given at the same ages (except at eighteen months) protects her against poliomyelitis.

It is important that the community's level of immunity to these diseases remains high—all children should be immunised to keep the remainder of the community healthy and to stop the spread of disease.

Immunisation is easy to obtain, effective and carries few risks, and is certainly less risky than contracting the diseases it protects against. Occasionally there are reactions to the whooping cough part of the immunisation programme, but most of these are mild—severe complications are rare. Whooping cough is a dangerous disease, and the decision not to immunise your child against whooping cough should not be made lightly or without the advice of your doctor. Giving your baby a dose of infant paracetamol at the time of immunisation reduces the risks of her developing a temperature. Ask your doctor about the correct dose for your baby.

If your baby has had any immunisations in the previous three weeks, or a blood transfusion in the last three months, a doctor needs to be informed before any injections are given. If your child has a temperature over 38 degrees Celsius (100.4°F), she should not have the injection until she is better.

If your baby vomits within two hours of having the syrup for poliomyelitis, the immunisation needs to be repeated. If your baby has a reaction to immunisation, such as a fever of 40.5 degrees Celsius (104.9°F), persistent screaming, vomiting or fits, you should inform your doctor immediately.

Haemophilus influenzae type b (Hib) is a life-threatening condition for children under five years, especially those between six and eighteen months of age. Before the introduction of a vaccine there were

10 to 20 deaths each year in Australia, and another 20 to 40 children had permanent problems following this condition. This condition includes meningitis (which is an infection of the membranes covering the spinal cord and brain), epiglottitis (an infection of the throat), cellulitis (an infection deep in the skin, usually around the face), septic arthritis (an infection of the joints) and pneumonia (an infection of the lungs). To prevent your baby getting this infection a course of injections can be given. There are two different schedules for this immunisation. One schedule is given at the same time as the first three Triple Antigen injections; at two, four, six and eighteen months. The second is given at two, four and twelve months. Your doctor will decide which schedule is best for your baby. What is important is that your baby is immunised against this serious condition.

It is normal for your baby to have a slight redness and swelling where the injection was given. She may also be miserable and not eat well for a couple of days after the injection. This is also normal.

Measles, mumps and rubella immunisation is given as a combined injection at twelve months of age. Measles is a highly contagious disease that can have complications for your baby. Immunisation helps reduce the risk of the community, especially children and, in the case of rubella, pregnant women, coming in contact with these diseases. It is possible to get a mild reaction such as a fine rash or fever approximately one week following the injection. The rash is not contagious, and using infant paracetamol under doctor's advice will reduce the fever.

If, for some reason, there is a delay at any stage of the immunisation schedule, it is not necessary to start the whole programme again. The course can be continued and adjustments made for future immunisations. Keep a record of your baby's immunisations for reference.

Hepatitis B is a serious condition which can lead to liver disease in adult life. Some community groups have a high incidence of carriers of hepatitis B, and it is possible that your baby will become infected. Some babies have a high risk of contracting this disease from their mothers. It is possible to have a blood test during pregnancy to determine whether the mother is a carrier of hepatitis B. To prevent the baby being infected, a course of injections can be given: the first injection is given soon after birth, the second at one or two months and the third at six months.

Tuberculosis immunisation ('BCG') is given to some babies of parents whose country of origin has a high level of tuberculosis. This injection is normally given soon after the birth of the baby. It causes a small sore on the arm where the injection is given, and the baby can have a little swelling under the arm, which may last a few weeks.

Minor ailments in newborn babies

Both **sneezing** and **hiccups** are normal in your small baby. Sneezing is her only method of clearing her nose, and with new smells and new clothing, most babies sneeze frequently. Your baby will do better without talcum powder, as it dries the skin and can also make her sneeze.

Hiccups are caused by the irregular contractions of the baby's immature diaphragm. This is common while your baby is feeding or when she has just finished a feed. This does not disturb her, and usually does not need any treatment. If it upsets you, just put her back on the breast for another minute or two; if you are formula feeding, give her about 30 mL (1 fl oz) of cooled boiled water. These measures are not usually necessary, however. Perhaps you can reassure yourself with the myth that the hiccups are a sign of growing!

Some small babies develop **sticky eyes**. This is caused by the fact that tears are not formed for the first three weeks of life, so that the eye is not washed as in older babies and adults. If the eye has a yellow discharge, it should be looked at by a doctor and treatment given as soon as possible. Occasionally babies have blocked tear ducts and this causes sticky, crusty eyes that may require eye massage. The baby should be looked at by a doctor to eliminate the possibility of infection.

Sticky eyes can also be bathed with salted water. Make up 300 mL (10 fl oz) of cooled boiled water and add 2.5 mL (half a teaspoon) of salt. Store it in a sterilised container in a cool, dark place. Make up a new solution every twenty-four hours. *Make sure you label this salty water well, and keep it away from your normal cooled boiled water, as your baby could become very sick if she swallows the salty water.*

Prickly heat is a condition that affects many babies in hot weather and in the hotter parts of Australia. It occurs around the neck and in the folds of skin, and also over the body in small babies. It is a fine, itchy rash of raised spots that in extreme cases can form blisters.

To treat prickly heat, try to keep your baby cool, and use a prickly heat powder or calamine lotion. Two teaspoons of sodium bicarbonate in your baby's bath will also help reduce the rash.

To keep your baby cool, dress her in only a singlet and a cloth nappy. Place her in the coolest area of the house — in the hallway or in the annexe if you live in a caravan. A bouncinette will allow the air to get to her skin on all sides. If you can afford to, use air-conditioning, even if only in one room. Otherwise, use fans. Overhead fans are more effective (and safer) than portable fans, as they circulate air better. Close your curtains to keep the house cool; having tinted windows can also help.

Take care that your baby does not become chilled; it may be necessary to dress her in loose clothing to prevent this.

If you place your baby under a tree for shade, make sure that sunlight is not filtering through onto her, and if you have to go out, make sure that she wears a cotton sunhat and that the pram hood and a light cloth shade her from the sun. Bathing her in the heat of the day will also help, and just before she goes to bed at night, to help her sleep. A short-haired lambskin helps keep her cool and absorbs the perspiration from her skin better than do cotton sheets. An unlined bassinette made of cane will also allow the air to flow around her body.

In extremely hot weather, babies **dehydrate** rapidly and need to have extra fluids. Mostly your baby will need a drink that is thirst-quenching rather than a feed. Cool boiled water is a good thirst-quencher for bottlefed babies, or breastfed babies who appear to be thirsty. If you are feeling thirsty, it's a good idea to offer the baby a drink as well.

Bowel motions

The first **bowel motion** of a baby usually consists entirely of meconium, and is passed during the first twenty-four hours of her life. Meconium is a sticky substance, dark green to black in colour. It can take several days for the bowel motions to change to a 'normal' consistency and colour.

There is a great variation between babies as to what is the normal consistency and colour of bowel motions. The type of milk used for feeding will influence the colour, odour and texture of the bowel motion. Breastfed babies' bowel motions are usually bright mustard-yellow in colour. The texture can be semi-formed to runny. They are usually less smelly than bottlefed babies' motions. The frequency and amount of bowel motion will vary greatly for the breastfed baby, from a small motion at every feed to an enormous one every seven days. If your baby has a bowel motion every seven days, you may find that she is unsettled and restless on the day prior to the motion.

It is rare that a breastfed baby becomes constipated. If your breastfed baby does not have a bowel motion after seven to ten days, it is probably worthwhile checking with your early childhood health nurse or doctor.

The bottlefed baby may pass a bowel motion at every feed or at one to two-day intervals. The bowel motion can be a pale yellow or greenish colour. It is usually of a paste-like texture and has an odour.

It is not normal for bowel motions to be very offensive, or green and watery. You should take your baby to the doctor immediately if they are, as this can mean that she has a germ in her bowel.

Changing your baby's nappy

Your baby will need to have a nappy change at least each feed time and sometimes between feeds if she is unsettled. When you change your baby, you will need some warm water or a wet warm washer. When you are out, you may choose to use a nappy change lotion, but avoid using commercial lotions on a baby who has any type of rash, as they will further irritate her skin. Wash well in the folds of your baby's skin. Wash her from front to back, to prevent infection of the vaginal area from the anus. With a boy, do not pull back the foreskin on the penis, as you may cause some damage.

Nappy liners are not essential items of equipment, but you may find these convenient, as they keep the greater part of bowel motions off the nappy and make nappies easier to wash. Disposable and cloth nappy liners are available. Disposable ones should not be flushed down the toilet; flush any bowel motion away, but dispose of the liner itself in the household garbage — check first to make sure that this is legal in your state. The initial cost of cloth liners can be expensive, depending on how many you buy, but if used as recommended by the manufacturer they can be effective in lowering the risk of nappy rash. Creams you use on your baby's bottom can block the pores of some cloth liners, reducing their capacity to draw moisture away into the nappy.

Washing nappies

Special care should be taken with your baby's nappies, as they are a potential source of infection. All new nappies should be washed prior to use. Two methods that can be used to wash nappies are described here.

Before **hot-water washing**, always remove as much of any bowel motion from the nappy as you can, and flush it down the toilet. Rinse the nappies in running water and place them in a bucket of plain water to soak until you are ready to wash them. Remember to have a tight-fitting lid on the nappy bucket.

Use the hot-water cycle on your washing machine, and the longest washing period available. Use pure soap powder, the residue of which is less likely to irritate your baby's skin than that of commercial laundry powders. Nappies should be rinsed well to remove all traces of soap. The addition of white vinegar to the final rinse (a tablespoon to each 500 mL, or 1 pint, of water) assists in neutralising any traces of ammonia that may be left in the nappies. Ammonia is formed by bacterial action on the urine, and has an unpleasant smell.

If you are using **nappy sterilising solution**, make it up as directed by the manufacturer. The bucket you use should have a tightly-fitting lid. Prepared solution and concentrated sterilising solution or powder should be stored out of the reach of small children.

Always remove any bowel motion and flush it down the toilet. You can rinse the nappies under running water before placing them in the bucket of solution. Leave them in the solution for the time recommended by the manufacturer, and change the solution as recommended. Rinse the nappies well to remove any trace of the sterilising solution.

The best method of **drying nappies** is in the sun. Give each nappy a shake to remove the wrinkles before pegging it onto the clothes line; this will make it easier to fold into shape later. Clothes dryers fluff up the nappies and make them soft and easier to fold, but have the disadvantage of removing fibres from the fabric, causing them to wear thin quickly.

Nail cutting

Some parents find cutting their baby's nails a little daunting at first. It is worthwhile investing in a pair of nail scissors specially designed with round-tipped blades for use with babies.

When your baby is small, it is often easier to cut her nails while she is sleeping, or you can have your partner or a friend nurse the baby while you cut the nails.

Hold your baby's fist and put out one finger at a time. Cut straight across the top of the nail. Take care not to cut the skin. The 'quick' in small babies grows right to the top of the nail, so tearing or biting the nail is not recommended.

Bathing your baby

Bathing your baby can be a frightening experience at first, but after a few attempts at bathing, you will probably find your confidence growing and your baby's enjoyment of the bath reassuring. Do not be disheartened if your baby cries; most babies cry initially when being put into or taken out of the bath because they feel insecure when not wrapped.

Bathing should be a relaxing time for you and your baby. If you are alone at home, take the phone off the hook to ensure that you are not interrupted. If you have another child, make sure you know where he is throughout the bathing time, and if you need to check on him, take the baby with you. You can often have the older child help you bathe the baby by passing you the things that you need.

The following technique is included as a guide only; the use of the oil for the creases of your baby's body is optional.

Preparation is the key to success. Have all the equipment that you will need ready. This will probably include:

- a small plastic bath
- a non-slip rubber mat for the bath, and another for the floor for you to kneel on
- non-perfumed mild soap, or bathing solution
- non-perfumed oil such as olive or almond, or sorbolene cream
- two washers or flannels
- a clean towel
- a clean nappy
- clean clothing
- a container for discarded cotton balls, and cotton tips and methylated spirits (if used) until the umbilical cord comes off and the umbilicus is healed.

There is no set time to bathe, but whenever you choose to, be sure that the room stays warm until you have finished and your baby is fully dressed, so that she does not become cold. Close the windows to keep out draughts, and use a heater in winter to keep the room warm.

Some parents find it easier when the baby is little to bathe her in the nursery area, because everything you need is probably already there and there are fewer hard and slippery surfaces than in the bathroom.

A new mother should not carry a full baby bath of water, and anyone lifting it should do so carefully, bending at the knees. It is better that the bath is filled using a smaller container or bucket carried to and from the tap, and emptied the same way.

Fill the bath three-quarters full with warm water, using cold water first and then adding hot water. Test the temperature of the water by splashing some on your inner arm, not your elbow or hand.

If you are using the main bath, run the cold water and then add the hot water. Finally, run the cold water again so that your baby will not burn herself if she touches the tap. This will develop safe habits for later, when you may be busy and less careful. If the tap rotates, move it out of the way.

FROM BIRTH TO THREE MONTHS

Do not undress your baby until everything is ready, and leave her nappy on until you have washed her face and hair. If her nappy is dirty, you will then be able to wash her nappy area immediately in the bathwater, without having to worry about keeping the water or your hands clean for her face and hair.

Wrap your baby firmly in the towel. Wash her face using a soft washer or flannel dipped in the bathwater. Do not use soap. Dry her face gently with the towel. Use some plain oil behind her ears; this moisturises any dry areas and helps remove any fluff that has collected there.

Place your baby on her back along the length of your arm, supporting her head with your hand. Pull her close to your chest and under your armpit, and wet her hair with the washer and clean bathwater. Return her to the bench and use a small amount of the soap to lather up her hair.

Talk to her when you are doing this, and massage her head gently and firmly. You will probably find that she likes this massage, and it will also help prevent her getting cradle cap. Do not be concerned about damaging her head by rubbing on the soft spot on top (the anterior fontanelle); this is made of cartilage, and if you rub with the flats of your fingers this will be quite safe.

When you have finished the massage, place your baby on her back under your arm and rinse off the soap in a backward direction, using the washer and taking care not to get soap in her eyes.

Return her to the bench and dry her hair with the corner of the towel, or with another towel if you prefer.

If you are using bathing solution, add it to the bath at this stage. Some solutions are drying or irritating for babies with sensitive skin, so test for this before immersing your baby in a bath of the solution.

Remove the nappy and apply oil to the creases of your baby's neck, underarms, elbows and wrists, under her knees and around the ankle area and the toes and fingers, and finally in the creases in the groin area. This will help to remove lint and fluff that has come off new clothing, or traces of creams in the groin area, and it prevents dryness, rashes and redness developing. If your baby has very dry skin, a non-perfumed oil may be used over the entire skin area before and after the bath.

After applying the oil, soap your baby, either in the bath or on the bench. Many new parents feel more secure soaping on the bench, and this allows you to concentrate on holding the baby securely once she is in the bath, without having to worry about soaping her.

When the soaping is finished, support your baby's head with the inside of your wrist and hold her upper arm securely in your fingers. Place your other hand under your baby's buttocks, and when you feel confident lower her into the bathwater gently, feet first. It is often helpful to move your baby from side to side slowly as you lower her, to get her used to the water. Lower her until all but her head is under water.

Talk to your baby while you are doing this, and try to have some eye contact with her. A lot of babies cry when initially placed in the bathwater. Check that the water is not too hot if your baby cries; even if it feels fine to you, if your baby turns red, the water is too hot. If the water temperature is definitely not the cause of the crying, be patient; many babies love the bath after the first few minutes.

Rinse your baby well, paying particular attention to creases and between fingers and toes. Wash the groin area well. Do not pull the foreskin back if your boy is not circumcised, as the skin is adhered until three or four years of age and need only be washed gently. Wipe baby girls gently from front to back with clean water and cottonwool.

Wash your baby's back by swapping your free hand for the one supporting the baby, moving the baby onto her stomach in the process. To ensure that her mouth remains out of the water, cup her cheek in the palm of your hand, supporting her chin with your little finger.

Wash your baby's creases well and rinse all the soap off before taking her from the bath. Immediately after lifting her out, wrap her tightly in the towel and give her a cuddle. This will usually calm her if she starts crying, and cuddles never go astray.

Dry her well, particularly her creases and groin area. If she has dry skin, reapply the oil. Use any cream necessary in the nappy area. Baby powder is not recommended, as it tends to dry out the skin and usually makes babies sneeze. Remove the wet towel and dress your baby.

Dress her in a singlet first, immediately followed by a nappy. When

SAFETY WHEN BATHING YOUR BABY

- Never leave your baby alone on a bench or table at any time.
- Always check the temperature of the water on the skin of your inner arm.
- Put the cold water in the bath before the hot water.
- Run cold water through the tap after you have been running hot water.
- Take care not to allow your baby to get cold.

dressing her, gather the clothing into a large circle and lift it over her face so as not to frighten her. Sleeves can also be gathered in this way, and your baby's hand held to guide it through long sleeves. Newborn and premature babies will require bootees unless it is an extremely hot day, as they have poor circulation. Check that long sleeves of inner clothing are pulled down under cardigans and jumpers, for warmth and to avoid constriction of your baby's arms.

Comb your baby's hair and, if she is still wakeful, just enjoy the time with her, talking and singing to her.

Enhancing development

When your baby is small you will not need a lot of toys or equipment to help her develop. Everything is new to her, from the feel of your clothing and the varying colours that you wear to the tone of your voice. Putting a few colourful toys in the bassinette and hanging a mobile over it will help her develop. (Remember, she will be able to see 20–30 cm (8–12") in front of her face.) Taking her for a walk outside and talking to her will help her get a feel for the world.

Changing her position and posture can also help her get used to her own body. When you are doing housework, talk or sing to her and move her from room to room with you. If she is unsettled, carry her about with you in a pouch. When she is calm, put her on a colourful bunny rug with a few toys. Remember to change her position from time to time and make sure that she is safe from animals and toddlers.

Remember to talk to your baby and give her lots of hugs. Playing with her fingers, hands, feet and toes will be enjoyable for both of you. Anything that makes you feel happy, content and loving towards your baby will be good for her, so relax and trust your instincts.

Safety

If you are travelling with your baby in a car, be sure to use an approved safety capsule. The lining should be the one that is provided with the capsule, as other liners will move in an accident and could allow your baby to slide from the capsule. If you are using a blanket, secure the capsule safety band around the baby and then place the blanket on top.

Take care never to place your baby in a position where she could fall. Do not leave her unattended at any time, either on the change table or on a bed, not even for a second.

Do not put your baby on a water bed. Small babies need to use their hands to lift up their heads so that they do not smother, and on a water bed there is nothing for them to push against, as the bed gives way to pressure.

See appendix I for general safety guidelines.

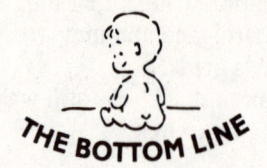

THE BOTTOM LINE

- Get to know your baby: she cannot be spoiled at this age, so hold her and cuddle her as much as you like.
- Be prepared to organise your household around your new baby's needs and her irregular schedule.
- Be flexible: try a few different methods of carrying out the basic skills of changing, bathing and entertaining your baby to see which suits you both best.
- Take care of your own physical and emotional needs: if you are not happy or well, your baby won't be either.
- Immunise your baby for her own safety and that of the community.
- Aim to have more good days than bad.
- Expect your baby to have a crying period of two to four hours every day.
- Use the 24-hour Parent Help Line if you need to.

CHAPTER 7

From three months to six months

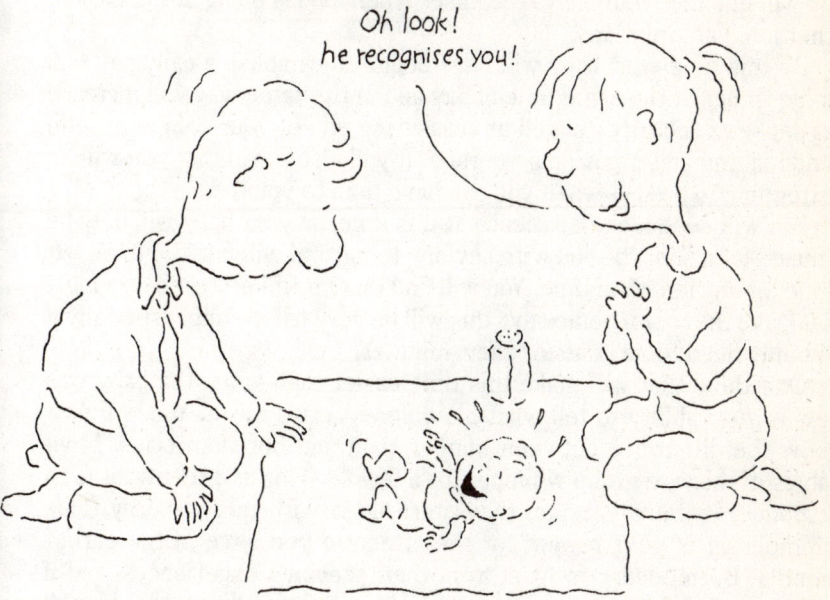

Oh look! he recognises you!

Development at three months
- Watches own hand movements
- Holds rattle placed in hand
- Focuses easily in all directions
- Vocalises when spoken to
- Coos and smiles easily
- Pleasurable response to familiar situations, such as bathing
- Follows moving person with eyes, especially when feeding

Average sleep
- 8–10 hours at night
- Wakeful during the day
- 2 day sleeps at least

Feeding
- 3–5 hourly feeding, about 5 feeds a day
- 150–180 mL (5–6 fl oz) per feed if formula fed
- Solids after about four months
- Offer breast or formula before solids at each feed, until six months

Weight gain
Steady at 150–200g (5–7 oz) per week

Immunisation
Second Triple Antigen, oral Sabin and Hib at four months.

Between four and six weeks, your baby will probably have begun to smile in response to your smiles and talking, and by three months he will most likely have developed a pattern of responding to both his parents, or to anybody he sees very regularly, with smiles, laughs and coos.

His curiosity about the world will also be noticeably greater than before. You will find that he is more alert, spending less time sleeping. Most babies love to be bathed and generally cooed over at this age, and you will find that your baby recognises when food is being prepared, and other familiar situations.

By this time your baby will have begun to establish a daily pattern. Doing things at the same time of day and in the same way will increase his sense of security, as well as reassuring you of your competence in handling him and organising yourself. It will also mean that you will be better able to predict when you can have time to yourself.

You will need a bit of patience at this time, as your baby will only be amused for a short period with any one thing, and will not like to be left alone for any length of time. You will find that he will protest by crying if you leave the room. Some days this will be very frustrating, especially if you only need to be gone for a few minutes.

One thing that will make this time easier than when the baby was new is your ability to tell what his different cries mean. You will now know the difference between hunger, pain and boredom cries. Most babies of this age group whimper for a few seconds and then wait for a response. If there is none, they start again with more energy. This whimpering is your reward for the attention you gave in the earlier months. Babies learn to trust from their previous experiences, and if you have given your baby attention before and met his needs, he will learn to wait for you for a short time.

Sleep

Your baby by now will usually sleep from the last feed at around 10 o'clock at night until about 5 o'clock in the morning, although this will vary with each baby and especially if you are breastfeeding. His sleeping patterns will change over the next few months, and he will be awake for longer periods in the daytime, and you may need to summon extra energy at this time.

Occasionally babies who were previously sleeping well at night go through periods of night waking. There are many causes of night waking, but the common ones for this age group are dealt with here.

By four months most babies have **outgrown their bassinettes** and

FROM THREE MONTHS TO SIX MONTHS

need to be moved into a cot. This is because they are growing bigger and moving more, and tend to hit the sides of the bassinette and wake themselves up.

See pages 23–4 for factors to note when buying or borrowing a cot. If you have venetian blinds, make sure that your baby cannot reach the cord from his cot, as there is a risk of him strangling or choking on the cord. When you are putting your baby down in his cot, always put the cot sides up and check the hinges before you leave him.

This age is often a good time to move your baby to a **separate room**, if you have not already done so. He is much more aware of his surroundings, is more easily wakened by noises and has much better vision than before. He will be very sociable, and a chat with you at two or three o'clock in the morning may be a very attractive idea for him, but may cost you and your partner some sleep. If you are not within easy access, he may drift off to sleep instead.

Waking at night **after a cold or after the second immunisation** is not uncommon. Your baby may be unsettled for one to three days after immunisation, although most babies will have few problems. You may find that you have to get up to him during this time, to change him or settle him or just to reassure him that you are there.

You may even want to bring him back to your own bed, although sleeping with a restless four-to-six-month-old is not advisable, as often you do not get much sleep. You may feel happier to have the baby near you during periods of night waking, however.

You can try moving the cot or bassinette closer to the bed as an alternative to sharing your bed with your baby. This avoids the problem of getting your baby back into the habit of sleeping in his cot or bassinette once the night-waking period is over. Most babies enjoy company, and it's lonely in your cot if you've become used to sleeping with mum or dad!

To help re-establish the sleeping pattern, get up to your baby if he is crying. Speak calmly and perhaps give him a small cuddle, but try not to lift him from his bassinette or cot. Being calm and touching him reassures him that you are nearby and still love him. You may have to do this for a few nights, but if you are consistent, his sleeping pattern will return.

Loss of the dummy can cause a baby to wake, as a small baby cannot replace his lost dummy. You have two options. You can continue to replace the dummy — if he is sleeping in your bedroom this is possible, though it does nothing for your own sleep. Your second option is to remove the dummy.

This stage is a good time to do this; as he grows older he will become more strongly attached to the dummy as a comforter. It is also harder to keep the dummy clean as your baby becomes more mobile.

During heatwaves or excessively cold nights babies may be disturbed and not sleep well. During a heatwave, dress your baby in a singlet and nappy and try to keep his room cool. Do not position a fan so that it blows directly on him, as he will lose heat rapidly. Take care that the fan is also out of his reach and not too close to the bedclothes. In very humid regions an overhead fan is better at circulating air than any other type of fan. Cooled boiled water can be given in these extreme times, if you think thirst is keeping your baby awake.

In extremely cold weather, do not overdress your baby, as this can be uncomfortable for him and cause heat rash. Bonnets, mittens and bootees will probably be needed.

Waking because of a wet nappy is occasionally a problem. You can solve it by using double nappies at night with flannel pilchers or pilcher products, preferably without plastic backing. A small amount of vaseline on your baby's skin will protect it from irritation.

Sleep disturbances **after a holiday or in a strange room** are more common after six months, but may be the cause of your baby's night waking at this age.

Most babies dribble from about four months of age, because their salivary glands are more mature, and because by this time they are able to put their hands (and anything in their hands!) into their mouths at will, stimulating the production of saliva. This is often mistaken for a sign of teething. The majority of babies teethe at about six months of age, and teething is not usually a cause of night waking until that time.

Feeding

Weaning, and the introduction of your baby to solid foods, are covered in chapters 12 and 14, but there are a few things to note about feeding babies of this age.

It is important not to start your baby on solid food too early, for a number of reasons. Your baby obtains all the nutrition he needs for growing in the first six months from either breastmilk or formula. The risk of him developing an allergy to some foods is higher during these early months. He is more likely to become constipated if he is eating a lot of solids and drinking less milk, and he may become unsettled and restless.

General guidelines for introducing your baby to solids are:

- Offer breastmilk or formula first, until your baby is six months old.
- Offer only small amounts of solid foods at first.
- Don't add sugar or salt to any foods you offer him, and steer clear of commercial baby foods containing added salt and sugar.
- Check for allergy with each new food you offer him, and allow three days before introducing another new food, so that if he reacts badly you will know which food has caused the problem.
- Fresh food is best — the greater proportion of what you offer him should be home-cooked.
- Remember that your tastebuds are mature; your baby will have much blander tastes than you.

Enhancing development

To enhance your baby's development at this time, give him floor play for as long as he seems to enjoy it. It is important and helpful for his development. It gives him an opportunity to exercise the muscles needed for normal growth and development.

Floor play is essential to allow your baby to learn how to roll over, which will happen in the next few months, and will help him gain strength and practice in sitting up, which he will be able to do, with support, by about six months. It also gives him the opportunity to experience new sights, sounds and textures, and to see the effects of his efforts. The use of baby walkers is not recommended for babies as they do not provide such experiences and encourage babies to walk on their toes. As accidents with walkers were common they are now banned from sale.

Place your baby on the floor; if you are doing housework, put him where he can see into the rooms you are working in. This will give both of you the ability to supervise each other!

If you do not have carpet, a small bunny rug or blanket will keep your baby off the floor. Having hard or cold floors is no excuse not to put your baby on the floor. The bunny rug also helps keep the floor clean, as by four months most babies are dribbling to some extent.

Place some toys within your baby's reach. These should be easy to grasp, brightly coloured and preferably washable. It is now possible to buy inexpensive small frames from which to hang toys.

You may also like to leave your baby without a nappy for a short time. This gives him a little more freedom of movement and also gives his nappy area some exposure to the air, which helps prevent nappy rash. Do not be surprised if your baby handles his genital area at this time. It is quite normal, does not hurt him and does not lead to any behavioural problems at a later stage.

A change of scenery can be fascinating for a small baby. Propping him up in his pram for a short period will allow him to see you and the room or the backyard from a different perspective; be careful that he is strapped in and cannot fall.

Your baby will probably love bathing by now, and you should try to make it a time of play as well as a practical exercise. You may wish to use the family bathtub now, to give him more space; a non-slip rubber mat in the bath is essential to prevent him slipping. Be careful when lifting your baby into and out of the bath; use a floor mat so that you do not slip if water has been splashed on the floor, and take care with your back. Bending your knees to lift your baby when he is small is a good habit to get into, so that when he grows bigger and heavier you will automatically pick him up correctly.

Your baby may now try to stand for a few seconds, and bounce up and down on your knee. This is normal; there is no truth in the myth that a baby who does this will be bowlegged. Encourage this leg strengthening activity, and your baby will probably laugh with delight.

Safety

In the next couple of months, your baby will learn to roll himself over. Be very careful from now on to put him only in positions from which he cannot possibly fall. Don't leave him unattended on the change table for even a second, or put him to sleep on a bed when you are visiting. *Falls are common at this age*, especially from couches, because even babies who cannot yet roll properly sometimes flip themselves over. If you have to leave your baby for any reason, place him on the floor.

Be careful if you have animals that both the baby and the animals are safe. Small babies still have a grasp reflex and have trouble letting go of anything they take hold of, and if this includes animal fur, tails or ears, your pet may react by scratching or biting your baby.

When travelling in the car, keep your baby in the capsule until he is six months old or weighs 9 kg (20 lb), when he should have sufficiently good head control to change over to a safety seat.

When you take your baby outside, be sure to dress him in a sunhat and long-sleeved clothing to protect him from direct sunlight. See appendix I for general safety guidelines.

FROM THREE MONTHS TO SIX MONTHS

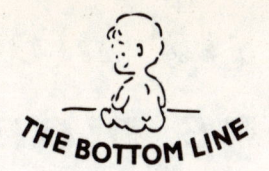

THE BOTTOM LINE

- Your baby's attachment to you will become obvious during this time. Enjoy being the most important people in his life!
- Keeping your baby entertained will start to occupy more of your time.
- At around four months, start introducing solids into your baby's diet.
- Be aware of the danger of your baby falling from change tables, beds and lounges.

CHAPTER 8

From six months to nine months

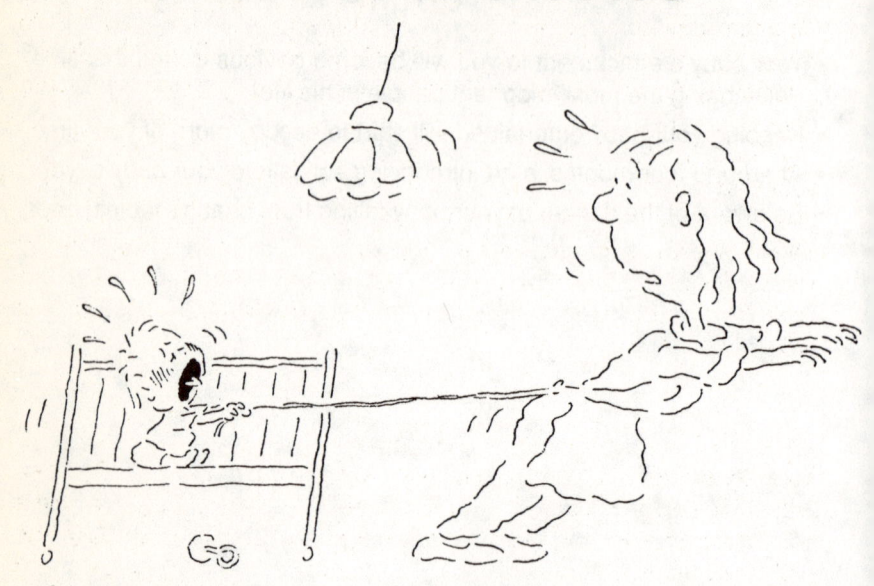

Development at six months
- Responds to own name
- Lifts arms to be picked up
- Puts feet to mouth
- Begins to imitate, for example, coughing for attention
- Friendly with strangers
- Shows response to different emotional tones of parents' voices
- Vocalises well, making such sounds as 'ma', 'da', 'goo'

Average sleep
- 12 hours at night
- 2 day sleeps

Feeding
- 2–3 meals a day
- Offer solid foods first, then breast or formula (200–240 mL, 7–8 fl oz) three to four times daily

Weight gains
By about five or six months your baby will be double her weight at birth, after which her weight gain will slow to half the previous rate. On average, this means that weight gains of about 100 g (3½ oz) per week are satisfactory. If your baby has been gaining smaller amounts on average in the first six months, these will halve also. These are approximate weight gains, and guides only, but if your baby is not gaining well or consistently, you should have her checked by a doctor to exclude the possibility of a physical cause.

Immunisation
Third Triple Antigen, oral Sabin and Hib at six months

FROM SIX MONTHS TO NINE MONTHS

Your six-month-old baby should continue to be friendly and sociable, very alert and responsive and aware of the world. As she comes closer to nine months, you may find that she becomes more cautious of people, both strangers and relatives. Often babies become more clinging towards the person who cares for them the majority of the time during this period. This can sometimes cause distress to grandparents or other relatives to whom the baby may have gone previously with ease and smiles. This is a normal part of development, and your baby will grow out of it by about twelve months.

This will be a tiring time for you or the person who gives most care to your baby, because she is difficult to settle with anyone else and this makes leaving her somewhat trying. It is normal to feel guilty at this time, but remember that this is an important learning experience for your baby. If left for a short period, she will learn that you will come back. Games like peek-a-boo and hiding toys under cloths will help her develop the idea of returning.

Sleeping

Your six-month-old baby will sleep for about twelve hours at night and will sleep better if she has two day sleeps. Day sleeps keep your baby content and prevent her becoming overtired and cranky. At this age she will sleep better in a cot and in her own room. She is now more easily disturbed by noises such as barking dogs, and can be woken more easily by normal household noises or by parents constantly checking on her as she sleeps.

The most common cause of disturbed sleep at this age is a change in routine, such as a holiday, or a change of environment. Waking as a reaction to immunisation, an illness, cold or teething is also common, and a routine needs to be reintroduced when these problems are resolved. Occasionally you may not notice signs of tiredness, such as eye-rubbing or whingeing, and your baby may then become overtired and be difficult to settle.

The fear of separation from you is beginning at this age and peaks at about nine months. You can help your baby settle at night with a short sleep routine with lots of hugs at the end, but be careful, as before, not to make the routine too involved as occasionally you may need to use it away from home.

If your baby wakes, go in and reassure her that you are there and resettle her. Some small soft toys in the bed can give her something to play with for a while when she wakes early in the morning.

Feeding

To feed a baby of six to nine months, you will need the following:

- highchair
- large plastic tablecloth
- small feeding bowl
- two shallow spoons with round, smooth edges
- large bib
- patience

If you have not already done so, this is the time to put your baby into a highchair to feed. When choosing a new highchair, buy one that is easy to clean, that is, with as few crevices as possible. The highchair should also have a wide base and a strap or a harness to keep your baby from falling. If you have a secondhand chair, check the hinges and joints for stability, and check the strap for wear and the buckle for safety. It is a good idea to place the highchair on a large plastic tablecloth, as food is spilled often when children are small. The highchair also should be away from dangerous objects, such as stoves, electric power cords or power points, that the baby might grab hold of.

Most children at this age need about 600 mL (21 fl oz) of milk and three meals a day. They are beginning to chew better, and are often more settled at mealtimes if they have something in their hands; giving your baby a spoon to hold while you feed her is a good idea.

Teething

Most babies get their first teeth by the age of six months, but some teethe much later. Some babies have no problems at all teething. Some medical professionals say that teething problems are a myth and that teething is as painless and worry-free as growing toenails, but those of us old enough to have wisdom teeth may not agree. Nor would many parents of small children who have suffered sleepless nights and miserable days every time a new tooth appears!

On the other hand, many people, even those who have had little experience with babies, will tell you that *any* problem you are experiencing with your child is due to teething. Teething is often blamed for problems that have quite another cause. Babies also place their hands, and anything else they can find, in their mouths at this age. This causes them to dribble quite a lot and is often mistaken for a sign of teething. For these reasons it is important to establish that teething is the problem before applying any of the advice in this section. If your baby's gums are pink rather than red and swollen, consider some other cause of her unsettled behaviour.

Stories of babies having difficulties if they do not cut teeth in the normal order ('cutting teeth on the cross') are unfounded.

Teething rings filled with water that are placed in the fridge to cool, or firm rubber rings or toys, may help soothe your baby's gums when she is teething. Make sure rings fit into your baby's hand and cannot break in her mouth. Check the seams to make sure that they are smooth, and if you are using a water-filled teether, check that it cannot split and allow the baby to swallow the water inside. You should not use secondhand water-filled teethers, as the previous user will have softened and weakened the plastic.

Some babies are soothed if their gums are massaged softly with a clean finger and boiled water or lemon juice.

Pieces of **apple, carrot or celery**, wrapped in a clean piece of cotton cloth or a handkerchief, can also be given to your baby for her to bite, but care should be taken that she is not left alone, as there is always a possibility of her choking.

Medications for teething should only be given after the doctor has decided that teething is the cause of your baby's distress. The directions should be followed carefully. **Teething gels and powders** should be used with caution as they often contain a local anaesthetic and aspirin, and should not be given with other oral pain relievers, such as paracetamol.

Fevers and loose bowel motions in small babies and children should always be checked by a doctor. Some babies and children have associated ear infections when they are teething. Paracetamol may be given for fevers, but it is not advisable to give aspirin to small babies or children. Medications that contain sedatives should only be given on medical advice and only with caution. For more information see chapter 17, 'Caring for your sick baby'.

Severe **rashes** need medical attention. It is common for a teething baby to get a rash on her chin, and sometimes on her chest as well, from the excessive saliva she produces. This can be avoided by putting a protective cream such as petroleum jelly on her chin and keeping her clothing dry by frequent changes of singlets or the use of a bib. You should not put your baby to bed with a bib on, however, for safety reasons.

SIGNS OF TEETHING

These symptoms are only a guide; babies and small children can suffer a combination of these or none at all.

- swollen gums
- excessive dribbling
- irritability
- flushed cheeks
- rash on chin and chest
- rash on buttocks
- redness around anal area
- biting
- waking at night
- pulling at ears
- temperature above 37.5°C (99°F)
- looser than usual bowel motions

These last three signs should *always* be checked by a medical professional.

Rashes on buttocks and around the anal area can be soothed by frequent washing and the use of a thick barrier cream such as zinc and castor oil, if no infection is present. Your baby can be left without a nappy for a short period to air the area (take care that she does not become cold), and you should avoid using pilchers while the rash persists. If the rash is severe or you are at all concerned, consult your doctor.

It is not necessary to wean your baby when she starts getting teeth. Many women continue to breastfeed for many months after their babies have teeth. Biting of the nipple often occurs when the breast has been emptied of milk, and it is normal for babies who are teething to bite anything that comes into contact with their mouths!

If you are breastfeeding and your baby is **biting**, it is usually only necessary to say 'no' firmly and remove her from the breast for a few minutes. Avoid rewarding her by reacting in an entertaining manner. If she bites you again when you return her to the breast, remove her again and do not re-offer her your breast until the next feed is due, or until a short period has elapsed.

Although teeth may take a few weeks to cut the gums, it is usually only for a day (and a night) or two that the major symptoms, such as a high temperature and wakefulness, occur. If these symptoms continue, you should have your baby checked by your doctor, as there is probably some other cause of them.

While your baby is teething, you may need to bring some coping

Dental care

Once your baby's teeth have appeared, you should start taking care of them. This can start with simple cleaning. No toothpaste is necessary. Once a day place your baby on your lap and with your finger lightly rub her gums for about a minute.

A small, soft-bristled toothbrush can be used, when your baby is used to the rubbing. After a while, a little fluoride toothpaste may be used. It will be necessary to clean your child's teeth for her until she is ten years of age; children do not have the co-ordination to do this for themselves until then.

Care should be taken that your child's diet does not contain too many sugary foods, as these can cause tooth decay. Sugary substances such as honey, jam or glycerine should not be placed on your baby's dummy for this reason. Cordials, juices and some juice substitutes contain varying amounts of sucrose (cane sugar), fructose (fruit sugar) and glucose. Your baby's intake of these sugars should be limited; reading the labels on these products will tell you which ones to avoid. Some brands that are labelled 'no sugar' actually contain large amounts of non-cane sugars such as fructose or glucose. Putting your baby to bed with sugary drinks can cause tooth decay.

As your baby becomes older the introduction of foods that require chewing into her diet will also help care for her teeth and gums. See chapter 14 on the introduction of solid foods.

Fluoride in the form of drops or tablets can be given to your child if it is not already present in the water supply or if you use a water filter. The addition of fluoride to the water supply has greatly reduced the incidence of tooth decay in children.

Small babies and children can be offered water rather than large quantities of juice or cordial. If juice is given, it is better that it is diluted with water. This gives fluoride, as well as lowering the amount of fruit sugar in contact with the teeth, and in the diet as a whole.

The care and protection of the primary teeth assists both in the quality of speech and in the spacing and appearance of the permanent teeth that follow. Regular checks by a dentist will be necessary after your baby reaches three or four years of age. It is often suggested that you take your toddler with you when you go to the dentist for a check-up to familiarise her with the environment and the procedure. If you are nervous of the dentist and anxious at these visits, this advice is not for you, as your toddler will probably be able to tell that you are not at ease and will become anxious herself.

Enhancing development

Your baby at this age can usually put either foot into her mouth and can roll successfully both to the left and to the right. You need to continue to allow her plenty of floor play. This is a good time to introduce her to a mirror, which will help her develop a sense of self.

Touching your baby's body, counting her toes and fingers and gentle massage also assist in her development. Blowing raspberries and making sounds encourages her to respond. When your baby begins crawling, she will love to clamber over you and your partner.

If your child is not vocalising by this age, she should be checked by a professional, at your local early childhood health centre or by your family doctor, to see that there is no problem with her hearing.

Toys for children of this age group should be small enough to fit in their small fists and durable enough to be put in their mouths with safety. Your baby will be able to transfer objects very successfully from one hand to another and also to let go. Colourful rattles are good toys. As with toys for all age groups, they need to be wiped over occasionally to keep them clean and free of most germs.

Your baby will enjoy dropping objects just to see them fall. To prevent your patience fraying after picking up toys the first twenty-odd times, tie them with a piece of string or cloth to the highchair or pram. This is especially helpful in the supermarket; it saves you hunting up and down the aisles for lost toys. The string should not be long enough to go round your baby's neck and choke her.

A large cloth with a drawstring sewn in around the edges enables you to put out your baby's toys on a soft, clean surface, and when play-time is over to pick them up in one go.

Don't put out all your baby's toys at once; give her a few at a time, and change them frequently. This will seem like a constant stream of new toys to your baby, who at this age only has a short memory. It is also worthwhile doing this with presents given to your baby at birthdays and other special times of the year.

Time in the fresh air is important, and walks in the pram can be an enjoyable experience for both parents and children. Be sure that you protect your baby from the sun with clothing and a hat, and give her some protection from the glare in the pram with a cover or umbrella.

Your baby at this age will enjoy music; whatever music you enjoy will be enjoyable to her. It is all a new experience. She will love to hear you sing, even if you can only do so out of tune; this may be the only chance you get to perform before a captive audience, so make the most of it!

Safety

Your baby will become even more mobile during the next three months. Check that you have childproofed your house, using the guide in appendix I, and try to be one step ahead of your baby's development. Going through your home on your knees will often help you locate dangers that you may not notice from adult height, and you will become particularly aware of the ease of access of most power points for small fingers. By now you should have installed either safety circuit breakers or power safety plugs. Moving your baby away from objects such as power points and indoor plants, or keeping dangerous objects away from her (your plants may do better outside for a few months), are the best safety techniques, combined with saying 'no' in a firm, loud voice.

The other most common mishaps for babies of this age are getting stuck under furniture and hitting their heads on the undersides of low tables they have rolled or crawled under.

Check any area where you put your baby down. Small, inquisitive babies can find all kinds of hazards, from small pins on the carpet to the tail of the family dog. Frequent vacuuming helps remove most of the tiny hazards from the floor, and supervision of animals will make your home safer for all concerned.

Use door barriers to keep your baby in one room, or at least out of dangerous areas, such as the kitchen or stairways.

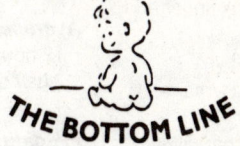

THE BOTTOM LINE

- Be prepared for clinging behaviour during this stage; it is a normal phase of development, which will pass.
- Enjoy introducing your baby to new foods — keep her meals simple and not fussy to prepare, for your own sake.
- Develop a dental care routine as soon as her first teeth appear.
- The possibilities for play will be much greater as your baby learns to move herself about (as will the potential for accidents!).
- Do not forget your baby's six-month immunisation.

CHAPTER 9

From nine months to one year

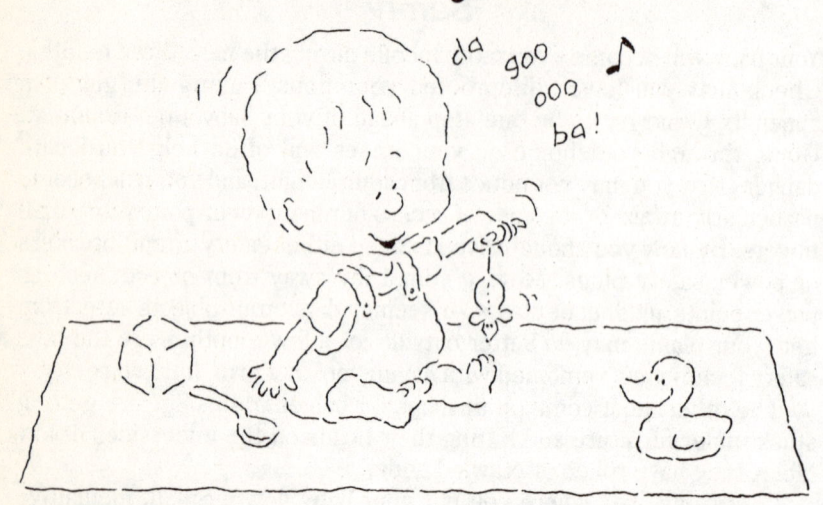

Development at nine months
- Can sit without support for 10–15 minutes
- When sitting, can lean forward without losing balance
- Waves bye-bye
- Able to clap hands
- Picks up objects using index finger and thumb
- Understands 'no' and 'bye-bye'
- Babbles tunefully: 'dad-dad', 'mam-mam', 'adaba'
- Strong attachment to main caregiver
- Becomes anxious when strangers approach

Development at twelve months
- Walks with one hand held, or holding onto furniture
- Uses both hands freely
- Picks up small objects
- Can say two or three words with meaning, as well as 'dada' and 'mama'
- Knows own name and responds immediately
- Drinks from a cup with a little assistance
- Likes to stay within sight and hearing of a parent
- Demonstrates affection towards familiar people

Average sleep
- 12 hours at night
- 2 day sleeps

Feeding
- 3 meals a day
- 3 breastfeeds or formula feeds (200–240 mL, 7–8 fl oz)

Weight gain
About 100 g (3 $\frac{1}{2}$ oz) per week

Immunisation
Measles, mumps and rubella at twelve months

FROM NINE MONTHS TO ONE YEAR

You will probably find that your nine-month-old baby will be very attached to you. He may cry when strangers approach and sometimes even when close relatives arrive. This can include grandparents who your baby may have previously gone to easily and without fuss. This is a normal part of childhood development, and your baby will be less shy by about twelve months.

If you are breastfeeding, the period from around seven months to around ten months is not a good time to wean, as this is the time when your baby is most clinging, and weaning may cause him more distress than at other times.

All babies have different temperaments, and some may have little trouble separating, while others may be very clinging. You may find any clinginess a little tiring as a parent, but it will soon pass, and your baby will return to being the sociable little person you remember.

If you do not have a regular baby-minder, it is better to wait until your baby is twelve months old before going back to work, if this is at all possible. Of course, there are many cases where it is not, and it is important that you give your baby lots of time in out-of-work hours.

Feeding

Your baby will now need three solid meals a day and three breastfeeds or formula feeds of approximately 200–240 mL (7–8 fl oz) per feed each day. Most meals that you prepare for yourself will be suitable for your baby to eat, unless they are highly spiced or contain large quantities of salt or sugar. Your baby, like yourself, will like food that has a variety of colours and textures.

It is important to give your baby food with a firmer texture at this age. This helps your baby to learn to chew, which will encourage the development of his facial muscles and the muscles necessary for speech. The food can be mashed with a fork, or fed to him in small pieces if it is soft enough for him to chew. You can also give him finger food after each meal.

Allow your baby to have a spoon to hold while you are feeding him. This will help him make the transition to feeding himself at a later stage. Your baby will also like to feel the food while he is eating, both in the bowl and in his mouth; this is perfectly normal and helps him learn about various textures. Make sure you have a wet washer handy to clean him with at the completion of the meal.

By twelve months, your baby will be able to drink from a cup with only a little help from you.

Sterilisation of bottles and teats

You will find that your baby tends to pick up and eat anything that is left on the floor, including pieces of fluff and crumbs and, if he is outside, leaves, sticks and dirt. This is quite normal. Because of this behaviour, you may feel that it is no longer necessary to sterilise equipment such as bottles and teats, but it is advisable to continue with sterilisation until your baby is twelve months old as a precautionary measure, as milk becomes contaminated very easily.

Sleep

Your baby will probably sleep for about twelve hours at night during this period, and should have at least two day sleeps. Often it is helpful to have a set day-sleep pattern for your baby. Consider the most reasonable time for your household, taking into account the timetables of each family member.

Your baby will sleep better at night if he has day sleeps; keeping him up during the day will not make him sleep better at night, but will tend to make him overtired, irritable and prone to fighting sleep at night. Look for signs of tiredness, such as yawning, rubbing of eyes or irritability, clinging or weepy behaviour; any or all of these are signs that your baby could do with a rest.

When you settle your baby to sleep, either in the day or at night, establishing some kind of ritual may help. Try not to make this too lengthy or involved; you should be able to carry it out while away from home, visiting or on holidays.

Before you begin, make sure that your baby is clean, dry, warm and not hungry or thirsty. It may be a good idea to put two nappies on your baby for sleeping, partly because by now your nappies will be wearing thin, but mainly because the volume of your baby's urine will have increased. Your baby may tend to kick off the blankets, so make sure that you dress him warmly, or, alternatively, put him in a sleeping bag made for babies.

The use of transitional objects as part of your going-to-sleep ritual can be helpful at this age. These are objects that children become attached to, that can help them separate from their parents. They can be a favourite teddy, a doll or a soft toy, a dummy or a piece of cloth. Any toy that you choose to be your baby's transitional object should be very durable, washable and able to be dried in the shortest possible time (for example, during your baby's afternoon nap).

Closing the curtains of your baby's room for the daytime nap, or turning off the main light at night, can be part of your ritual. Often small children sleep better with a small night light.

Say goodnight to your baby, give him a cuddle and a kiss, tell him that this is sleep time and leave the room. Most babies will settle easily, but if your baby cries, wait for a couple of minutes. Often he will settle himself if you do not go back in immediately.

Occasionally babies have problems putting themselves to sleep. Your baby may have been sick, had a cold or a recent immunisation, or you may have been on holidays or for some reason unable to let your baby cry. This sometimes happens if your partner works shift work and needs to sleep at odd times.

Comfort settling

Make sure that your baby is not sick and that you have back-up support before trying any method of comfort settling; it helps to try any new system at the weekend, when both you and your partner can be involved. It is also helpful to tell your neighbours what you are doing if they are likely to be disturbed by your baby's crying.

Try to settle your baby with a cuddle and a kiss. If he continues to cry, try the following method of comfort settling. Leave him for a few minutes, five minutes if possible. If you have not left your baby before, you will find this a little difficult, and some babies will be very distressed to be left in this way. Try not to be too disturbed by your baby's crying, but allow yourself to go back in if the crying is really distressing you. If the stress of listening is too much for you, it may help for you to close the bedroom door and go to the other end of the house or flat, or even outside, for the five minutes' waiting time. If you are having problems leaving your baby to cry, enlist the help of your partner or a friend.

If your baby is still crying after five minutes, go back in, make sure that he is safe and give him a cuddle to reassure him that you are near. Wait until his crying has eased, then put him back down and tuck him in again. Try not to let him go to sleep on your shoulder, as this will not get him used to the idea of settling himself to sleep. You can pat him gently to help him calm down. When you have tucked your baby in, say goodnight again and leave the room.

You may have to do this a few times, and your baby may cry each time you leave the room, but try to console yourself with the knowledge that he is safe, and wait no longer than ten minutes each time before you go back in. Your baby will eventually get the idea that bed is for sleeping.

If this method clearly is not working, and both you and your baby are becoming very distressed, you may wish to settle him using your usual method and try again later.

If you are having particular problems settling your baby, check with your local early childhood health nurse or your family doctor.

Speech

Between nine and twelve months your baby will begin to make more recognisable sounds, such as 'mam-mam', 'dad-dad' or 'ta-ta'. By about twelve months he will be able to use two or three words with meaning. He will shout for attention and imitate sounds that you make. He will recognise and quickly respond to his own name by twelve months. Encourage his attempts to speak by talking back and responding to him, and make this a learning experience for both of you.

Shoes

Your baby will be more comfortable barefooted inside the house when he is first learning to walk. His own small feet give him better grip and more stability than shoes would. Once he is walking outside, you will need to buy him some shoes.

Shoes should:

- be well-fitting and broad enough not to cramp the feet. (When putting your child's shoes on, check that his socks fit well and do not form any ridges between the shoe and the feet;
- be made of leather, preferably, because leather breathes naturally. If you are using vinyl or plastic shoes, make holes along the sides for ventilation;
- have an adjustable strap over the arch of the foot;
- have a supportive heel with no hard seams;
- have a flexible sole. If the sole is smooth, scuff it on a rough surface, such as cement, so that it provides better grip;
- have enough room to fit the feet. If you cannot take your baby with you when shopping for shoes, cut a strip of cardboard about 2 cm (1") wide and the length of your child's foot, adding a centimetre for toe room, and take it with you.

Enhancing development

Time on the floor is important at this stage, so that your baby can develop good muscle tone and co-ordination. It also helps him develop eye-hand co-ordination, vision and concepts of space and cause and effect.

Crawling is usually well under way by nine months, and between ten and twelve months your baby will probably learn to pull himself into a standing position using the furniture. When he first manages this, he will be unable to sit down again, and you will have to help him for a while. Be sure that all the furniture he is likely to take hold of is stable, and that any sharp corners are covered so that he cannot hurt himself if he falls against them.

If your child is a 'bottom shuffler', that is, if he sits on his bottom to move himself along rather than crawling, do not be concerned. Bottom shufflers eventually learn to walk just as crawlers do, and their shuffling does not affect their physical development in any way.

Children are natural learners, and will develop good muscles and intellectual skills if given the opportunity, unless they have some developmental delay, when they will need extra encouragement.

Your baby should be given the chance to practise crawling and moving himself around on the floor.

Attendance at playgroup can give you and your baby some opportunities to mix with other parents and babies. There are now all kinds of organised activities for babies; kindy gyms and exercise classes are some of these. If you are considering attending one of these, it is worthwhile checking that the co-ordinator has adequate training, such as physiotherapy qualifications, or has undertaken an approved fitness leader's course for children under five years of age, as there are exercises that can be harmful for small babies.

Organised activities are not the only way to encourage babies' development. You can do so at home, at no cost, by giving your baby varied opportunities and changes of scenery and position. A daily walk can give him new experiences and fresh air at the same time. Make sure that he is protected from the sun or wind with adequate clothing and a hat. Wear a hat yourself; your baby will soon learn that it is natural to wear a hat in the sun or wind.

If the weather keeps you indoors, make obstacle courses for him with the furniture, for a change. Don't forget to use the mirror that you introduced when your baby was smaller; babies love to look at themselves at any age. Make sure that the mirror is sturdy and will not shatter when dropped or thrown against a hard surface.

Toys also enhance development for this age group: suitable toys are colourful soft toys such as teddies and dolls and animals, large blocks, push and pull toys, colourful balls and sturdy cardboard boxes.

Make sure that these toys are safe, as your baby will inevitably place them in his mouth. They should be washable and well made, with no small parts (such as the button eyes of teddies) that can come off with sustained pulling, chewing or other abuse. They should not be too heavy, and the seams on teddies and other soft toys should be strong.

A large blanket on the floor to spread the toys out on will help keep some of them in the one area. When your child has finished playing just take the four corners and tie them together until next time. This will save you packing and unpacking toys.

Plastic kitchen articles make great toys. Keep them in a cupboard in the kitchen that is easily accessible to your child.

You can leave some toys in the cot for your baby to play with on waking. Be sure that they are not large enough for him to stand on and fall from the cot.

There are government, municipal and private toy libraries available in some states. These provide a wide variety of toys; some toy libraries are free and others charge a small borrowing fee. These allow your child to have a variety of toys without the expense of buying them all.

Playing games such as peek-a-boo helps your child develop the concept of permanence, and pat-a-cake gives him an early introduction to his body parts and helps develop co-ordination. Leaving the room and then returning immediately also helps your child to know and trust that you will return.

Your baby will like music, and will probably 'sing' by the age of twelve months. Dancing with your baby will also be enjoyable for both of you whether he stands on the floor or is carried around.

If your baby is playing contentedly alone, do not disturb his play; this helps him separate from you and become a little more independent. This also applies when your baby wakes in the morning or at other times after a sleep; don't go to him straight away if he is just lying quietly or playing by himself.

By twelve months of age your baby will be able to do some things on request, such as giving a toy or a cuddle.

Safety

Using appendix I on safety as a guide, check your house again for potential hazards, which will be multiplied greatly during this stage as

FROM NINE MONTHS TO ONE YEAR

your baby moves around more, and decide now, with your partner, which items your baby may touch and which items you are going to have to keep out of his reach. Be sure about your choice, because you will have to be consistent for the next few years. It is sometimes easier to remove items than to continually say 'no'.

Make sure you have gates at the tops and bottoms of stairs. Door barriers are also helpful now that your baby is more mobile. These are easily erected and movable from room to room. Most are low enough for an adult to step over with little trouble.

Replace your tablecloths with placemats while your baby is small, and place all hot foods in the centre of the table.

Do not drink a hot cup of tea or coffee within reach of your baby.

Make sure that your animals are safe from your baby, and vice versa. Feed your animals away from the baby, and do not let him play in their sleeping baskets.

Ensure that your baby's cot is not close to a blind or venetian cord, as this introduces a risk of strangling.

Keep a supply of long-life milk in the refrigerator if your area is often cut off by the weather. Also have a well-stocked first aid kit and a medicine cabinet with infant paracetamol, antiseptic lotion and a few medications for any conditions that your baby regularly suffers from, in case of isolation. Have emergency numbers handy in case you need medical help, and know how to use all the equipment in your kit.

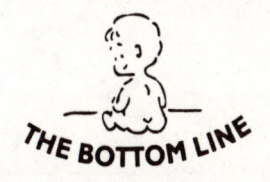

THE BOTTOM LINE

- Be prepared for mealtime messes — with plastic floor-coverings, a wash-cloth and, occasionally, a camera!
- Develop a regular, simple going-to-sleep ritual, for your baby's sense of security.
- Talk and read to your baby to encourage him to talk.
- Plenty of varied playtime will develop his muscle tone and his mind.
- Don't forget your baby's measles, mumps and rubella immunisation at twelve months.

Feeding Your Baby

CHAPTER 10

Breastfeeding

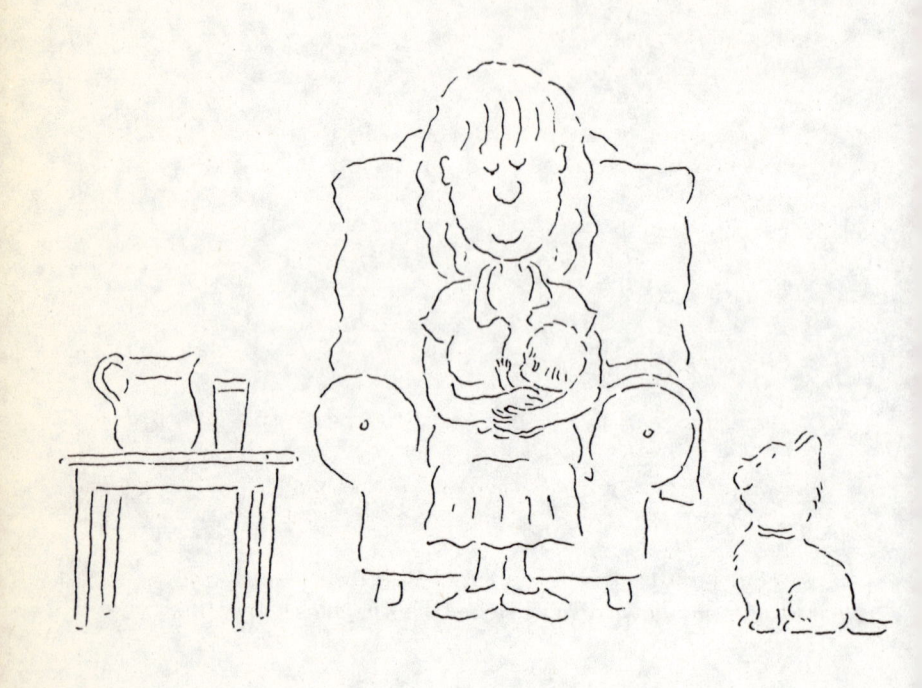

Breastfeeding has enjoyed a resurgence in the past decade, after a long period of unpopularity, and there are many good books entirely devoted to breastfeeding. In this chapter we give an overview of breastfeeding techniques, as well as some simple suggestions that may help mothers make the most of their natural ability to feed their babies.

For new parents, the pressure to fully breastfeed their baby may be very strong. A combination of breastfeeding and bottlefeeding can also work well if you are returning to work, if your milk supply is inadequate or if you need some time out from fully breastfeeding. If you are not happy fully breastfeeding, explore all your options before you decide to wean completely.

How breastmilk is made

Preparation to produce breastmilk starts to occur during pregnancy. There is a noticeable growth of breast tissue, increased sensation and change in the colour of the nipple and areola (the dark area that surrounds the nipple). The increase in the size of the breasts is due to the development of secretory tissue and alveoli, clusters of little sacs where the milk is made and stored.

The two main hormones for milk production are prolactin and oxytocin. Prolactin is produced in the anterior pituitary gland; its main function is to produce colostrum and milk. Prolactin levels rise steadily during pregnancy, but milk production is inhibited by the placental hormones progesterone and oestrogen.

By the fifth or sixth month of pregnancy there is a small quantity of colostrum in the breasts, which remains until a short period after delivery. Colostrum is a yellowish, sticky fluid, higher in nutritional value than normal breastmilk. Its other important property is that it protects the baby against infection.

Once the placenta has been delivered, the levels of progesterone and oestrogen fall, allowing the prolactin to stimulate milk production. This can take from forty-eight to seventy-two hours (though in some women it can take longer), during which time there is a transition from colostrum to breastmilk.

Oxytocin is stored in the posterior pituitary gland. When it is released, a letting-down of milk occurs. This enables stored milk to drain into the lactiferous sinuses. There are between ten and fifteen of these, and they lie behind the nipple. The rhythmical pressure of the baby's tongue can now remove the milk.

The 'let-down reflex' (that is, the release of oxytocin) is mainly stimulated by your baby's sucking, but the sight, thought or sound of a baby may produce this reflex. The let-down reflex may cause physical discomfort in some women, while others may not be even aware that it is happening.

The advantages and composition of breastmilk

Human breastmilk is the ideal milk for human babies. It is nutritionally balanced to suit your baby, and changes in composition to suit each stage of her growth. It provides protein mainly in the form of easily-digested whey curd. It helps protect your baby from infection, and the intensity of allergies is lessened, so your baby's body systems can mature before being challenged by foreign proteins.

Breastmilk is convenient and always at the right temperature. Your baby is able to regulate the quantity of milk she takes to meet her current needs. Breastfed babies are unlikely to become constipated, and their bowel motions are less offensive. And finally, breastfeeding helps the uterus return more rapidly to its normal size after the delivery of your baby.

Breastmilk is a constantly changing, living fluid. It changes in composition and quantity from feed to feed.

Breastmilk undergoes a transition from being entirely colostrum, through being a colostrum and breastmilk mix (which will appear rich and creamy), to mature breastmilk (which looks watery and thin). These changes take many weeks to occur, and other, more subtle changes may be noticed.

There is a difference between the milk your baby receives at the beginning and the end of each feed. The foremilk, which comes first, has a high proportion of lactose (sugar of milk). As the feed progresses, the milk changes, and at the end (the hindmilk) has a higher proportion of fats.

Lactose causes rapid gastric emptying, so if the baby receives only foremilk she may have frequent, explosive bowel motions and be generally unsettled. The high fat levels in hindmilk will help your baby to be more settled by slowing down her gastric emptying.

There was an emphasis in the past on babies gaining large quantities of milk by having them take milk from both breasts at each feed, but recent research has shown it to be more important for them to be left on a breast to gain the smaller quantities of hindmilk. This may mean feeding on one breast only at some feeds. Take care to check your other breast and offer it first at the next feed. Express for comfort if necessary. The best indicator of whether the breast has been emptied is if your breast feels empty or soft at the end of a feed. If after a few weeks your baby is taking more than forty minutes per feed it would be worthwhile asking your early childhood nurse to assess your baby's suck to check if it is efficient. Some babies only feed for ten minutes and that is fine.

Breast care

Caring for your breasts is an important part of breastfeeding. Start regularly examining your breasts so that you can detect any changes that occur, such as lumps or infections. (All women should make breast

BREASTFEEDING

examination a monthly activity as a matter of course, to detect early signs of breast cancer.)

When you are about four months pregnant, you may find it is more comfortable to start wearing a well-fitted, supportive maternity bra. This bra should have:

- no areas of constriction or pressure. Open the bra as if you are feeding to check whether there are areas of pressure that may restrict the drainage of your breasts;
- cotton sides and wide, non-stretch straps;
- easy openings. Remember, you will have to manage this while holding your baby;
- room to grow once you start to lactate. Lean forward to ensure that your breasts fill the bra cups before adjusting the straps. This will allow the best possible chance of adequate support.

Test the bra for comfort by sitting down while you are wearing it. As your pregnancy progresses, you may find it more comfortable to sleep in a bra at night. It is worth investing in only two maternity bras during pregnancy, in case you need to change bra sizes once you start to lactate. After you have the baby you will need at least three maternity bras: one to wear, a spare bra in case of soiling and one in the laundry.

The midwife or doctor should assist you in assessing the condition of your nipples. If they are flat or inverted, you can try to gently roll and extend them between your thumb and forefinger at bath time, though this may be of minimal assistance. If you have a history of miscarriages, avoid nipple stimulation as this can cause the uterus to contract.

Regular, short periods of exposure to warm air are advised (five to ten minutes only) to dry out and soothe sore nipples, as are daily showers and avoiding the use of soap, spirits or harsh towelling on your nipples, as these can remove the natural oil. It is not necessary, or recommended, for you to express colostrum prior to your baby's birth.

No special preparation is needed before you offer your baby the breast. The use of creams or lotions on the nipples is not recommended as a routine measure. If you have applied a cream or lotion to the nipple, gently wash it off with water before feeding your baby. At the completion of a feed, express a few drops of breastmilk and spread it over the nipple; its high fat content acts as a healing agent, with the added advantage of being an anti-infective agent.

Care of yourself while breastfeeding

Fulfilling the emotional and physical needs of new parents is of great importance, but the breastfeeding woman has additional physical demands placed on her by providing milk for the baby.

A positive, relaxed attitude towards your ability to breastfeed is the key to success. However, you will also need to take care of your physical health. A well-balanced **diet** is essential. While you are breastfeeding, you may find that your hunger increases dramatically. The exact amount of food you will need is dependent on how active you are, and at what stage of lactation. General guidelines on a healthy diet are given on page 173.

You should take great care with your diet. Avoid dieting and don't eliminate whole food groups, such as dairy products. It is important to get expert advice about eliminating foods from your diet, so that substitutes of equivalent nutritional value can be introduced.

Sufficient **fluid** intake is also very important — drink whenever you are thirsty (have a drink at hand while you are breastfeeding). Excessive fluid intake will not result in an excessive milk supply. Keep your intake of **coffee, tea and soft drinks containing caffeine** to a minimum, or reduce the strength of the coffee or tea you drink, as the caffeine is passed on to the baby through breastmilk and may cause your baby to be irritable and unsettled. Limit your intake of sugar and fatty foods, as they are of little nutritional value. **Alcohol** consumption and smoking should be avoided. **Nicotine** and alcohol can inhibit the let-down reflex. In addition, nicotine can reduce the amount of breastmilk that is produced.

CLOTHING FOR BREASTFEEDING

Your clothing needs may vary slightly from normal while you are breastfeeding. You will quickly learn to identify clothes that are easy to wash, and that provide easy access to your breasts and some degree of privacy if you are feeding in public. Clothing with a button opening up the front is useful for feeding at home, while tops that you can untuck and put the baby underneath are useful if you are concerned about privacy when feeding away from home or in front of visitors. Clothing made of patterned material is less likely to show up breastmilk stains than plain-coloured clothing. Many women find a lightweight poncho or shawl useful, as it provides privacy and helps to calm the easily distracted baby of six months or older.

The use of **medication** should be restricted to the absolute minimum. Always check with your doctor, pharmacist, or poisons information service to make sure that any medication you take cannot harm your baby.

Make sure you can take **time out** from looking after the baby for activities you enjoy, and have regular daily **exercise**. Adequate **sleep** is another essential for breastfeeding women. Accept offers of help with housework or childminding from friends and relatives.

Establishing breastfeeding

It is important to breastfeed your new baby as soon as possible after her birth. Ideally this first feed should occur soon after delivery, but if there have been difficulties with your baby or yourself this may not be possible.

Do not be overly concerned about establishing your breastfeeding, as regular expression (every three or four hours) or using an electric or hand pump during any period of separation will initiate and maintain your milk supply until you are able to put your baby to the breast. Always finish with several minutes of hand expression for extra stimulation. (See pages 138–9 for directions on expressing breastmilk.) It is common for your breastmilk supply to decrease during this period, but an increase in breastmilk will occur once your baby is sucking regularly at the breast, as a baby's sucking is the most efficient means of expressing.

Many women with premature or ill babies are able to initiate and maintain lactation for many months, until their babies are well enough to be breastfed, expressing and storing their breastmilk so that it can be fed through a bottle or tube to their babies by themselves or the nursing staff. Breastmilk is particularly good for an unwell baby, as it is easy to digest.

Breastfed babies should be allowed to regulate their own feeds; trying to be too highly organised is a recipe for failure. Most babies settle into a pattern of feeding every two to five hours if they are allowed to control their own feeding time at the breast and are positioned correctly, and if their mothers are feeling relaxed and enjoying breastfeeding. Unrestricted and efficient sucking by the baby results in successful breastfeeding for the majority of women.

Night feeds are an important part of maintaining an adequate supply of breastmilk; do not try to eliminate this feed too early. It is normal for night feeds to continue for at least three months, and some babies and their mothers continue for many months longer. Try to enjoy night feeds; they can be a special time with your baby, as there are no other pressures on you at this quiet time. Before going to bed each night, arrange your nappy-changing equipment so that it is close at hand. Have a shawl or light rug handy to throw over your shoulders while you feed, and a comfortable chair in the bedroom or in the most convenient room. The room should be a comfortable temperature; you may need to set up a heater to keep you warm during night feeds in winter. The hormone prolactin that is released when breastfeeding can assist you to go straight back to sleep.

Positioning yourself and your baby

When breastfeeding, make sure you are in a comfortable position. It is all right to change this position during the feed if you need to. Some women find it more comfortable to feed lying on one side in the early days after delivery, though it may be more difficult to attach your baby to the breast. The use of lots of pillows to support your back and the baby may help.

Your baby's face should be facing directly at the nipple, her chest facing your chest. Stimulate (tease) her mouth with your nipple. When she starts to open her mouth, wait a moment until it is as wide as possible, then quickly bring her to the breast. Use your free hand to support your baby's shoulders rather than her head.

She should be attached to the breast, not just to the nipple. Her bottom lip should take in most of the areola and will curl outward. If you feel any pain when she sucks, or your nipple becomes tender, the baby's positioning should be checked.

You will need to bring your baby in close to your own body. It is usually not necessary to depress your breast with your finger to assist your baby's breathing; with the above positioning she should be able to breathe without assistance. Depressing the breast will alter the baby's position, place extra stress on the nipple and interrupt the flow of milk through the depressed part of the breast.

Your baby's sucking should be rhythmical, with no sign of stress. She will pause for short periods, then resume sucking. Try not to limit your baby's sucking time; allow her to take herself off the breast. This usually occurs twenty to thirty minutes after the commencement of a feed, when she has fallen asleep. Some babies feed for longer or shorter periods. The baby may sometimes feed from one breast only at each feed, especially in the first few weeks, but you may need to offer the second breast if she is still sucking and you are concerned that she is still hungry. Alternate breasts at each feed—if you started with the right breast last feed, offer the left breast first at this feed. A small safety pin on your bra

BREASTFEEDING

can help you remember which side you fed from last time. Practise checking your breasts at the beginning, middle and end of a feed to learn the different feeling at various times during the feed.

As the feed nears completion your baby may appear to be asleep. However it is impossible for your baby to maintain a negative pressure (suction that has to be released) on the breast if she is asleep. Many babies wait with their eyes closed for another let down of milk. If you need to release your baby from your breast, gently slip your little finger between the baby's gums to break the suction (keep the nail of this finger short to avoid hurting the baby's mouth), and remove the nipple from her mouth.

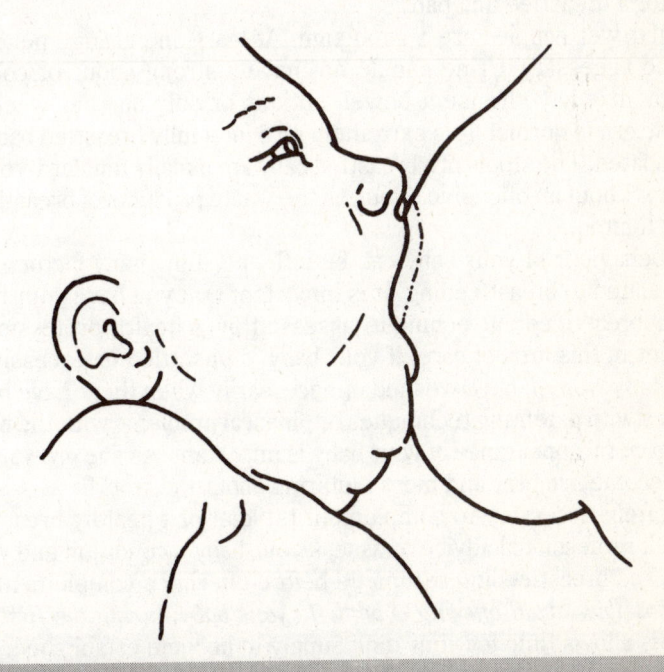

CHECKLIST FOR CORRECT POSITIONING

- Baby's mouth will be wide open with lower lip curled outward
- Baby facing front-on to the breast
- Baby tucked well in to your body
- No nipple pain when baby sucks
- Rhythmical sucking pattern with occasional pauses.

Is my baby getting enough milk?

One of the greatest concerns for breastfeeding parents is whether their baby is getting enough milk for her needs. The best guide you can use is your baby's behaviour and appearance. The early child health nurse or your local doctor will help you identify any problems.

Newborn babies normally lose weight in the first days after birth. During the second week your baby will probably regain this weight and return to her birth weight. At first, she will be weighed on a weekly basis when you visit the early childhood health nurse. You can expect these weight gains to be irregular; one week your baby may gain very little weight, the next she may have put on a great deal of weight. This is quite normal for a breastfeeding baby.

Regular wet nappies are a good sign. At least one change per feed should be necessary. Urine should not have a strong odour or colour. Your baby may have frequent bowel motions or only one per week — either pattern is normal. It is extremely rare for a fully breastfed baby to be constipated. The stools of a breastfed baby are usually mustard-yellow in colour without an offensive odour, as the waste products of breastmilk are very limited.

The behaviour of your baby can be influenced by many factors that are not related to breastfeeding. It is important that you have your baby and your breastfeeding technique assessed by a health professional, competent in this area of care, if your baby is unsettled or excessively sleepy. Many women have weaned unnecessarily when there have been difficulties with parenting techniques or physical problems with the baby.

The general appearance of your baby is important. As she grows, she should become brighter and more inquiring about the world.

It is rarely necessary to complement the diet of a healthy breastfed baby. Seek professional advice to assess your baby's condition and your lactation and breastfeeding technique before offering a complementary feed. *If possible, avoid offering a bottle to your baby during the first six weeks;* this allows time for your milk supply to become established.

If it becomes necessary to offer a complementary feed of formula, always offer it after the breastfeed, and limit the amount of formula given. It is rarely necessary to offer a complementary feed of more than 60 mL (2 fl oz); try to offer a complement only at times when your milk supply is low — for example, this may be at the afternoon and evening feeds. You may find it possible to express milk after each morning feed and give your baby this at the afternoon or evening feeds. After about ten to fourteen days many women worry about their supply as they have lost the 'full feeling', however this is due to the withdrawal of the increased vascular supply.

Breastfeeding after a caesarean section

Many women choose to breastfeed after they have had a caesarean section to deliver their baby. The time lapse between delivery and when you are able to offer your breast to your baby for the first time will be dependent on several things: the type of anaesthetic (general or epidural); your doctor's advice; and your physical condition and your baby's.

There are several positions you can use to feed your baby. You will probably need help in finding a position that feels comfortable, and it is important that you ask for help in changing positions if you become uncomfortable during the feed. Boomerang pillows or pillows placed under your arms to take the weight of your baby may be helpful. The positions that are usually suggested are:

- lying on your side with your baby resting on a pillow beside you;
- 'twin' fashion — the baby's body and legs are positioned underneath your arm, supported on a pillow;
- sitting up in a chair, with your arms supported by pillows, and a pillow on your lap to help protect your wound. A footstool to rest your legs on will take any strain from your abdomen. If you are resting your baby on a pillow, make sure that the pillow is protected with a towel.

Whatever position you choose, make sure you are comfortable. Rest as much as possible in the first weeks after the baby is born. It is important that you give your body time to heal.

Breastfeeding more than one baby

Many women successfully breastfeed their twins, triplets or quadruplets, fully or partially. This will take a little more effort, and at first you will need lots of support from other people so that you can obtain adquate rest. Do not be concerned if you need to complement your breastmilk supply with bottlefeeds as this is perfectly normal when you are feeding more than one baby.

The position and method you choose to use when feeding your babies will depend on how comfortable and confident you feel about handling your babies. You may find it easier to breastfeed each baby separately at first.

As your confidence grows, you may choose to breastfeed your babies two at a time. There are several points to remember:

- Alternate the breast you offer each baby at each feed, to stimulate an even supply of milk if one of your babies has a stronger suck than the other.
- Do not swap the babies around halfway through a feed, as one of your babies may miss out on a proportion of the hindmilk.
- Positioning the babies twin fashion (with their bodies underneath your arms, supported on pillows) is the usual method of feeding when they are little. Make sure that they are positioned correctly (see checklist on page 133).
- If you have more than two babies you may need to alternate their feeding at the breast with a bottle at other feeds. You should try to offer all the babies an equal time at the breast, keeping a notepad and pen by your chair or bed to help you keep track of who had the last breastfeed.

Your local early childhood health nurse may be able to visit you at home to give you support and advice about the care and feeding of your babies, as well as your own physical and emotional needs. The Multiple Birth Association also offers support, advice and equipment for rental.

Breastfeeding a premature or sick baby

Having a premature or sick baby can be very distressing for parents. If you have planned to breastfeed, don't give up the idea, as feeding breastmilk to your baby can be a positive step in helping her development and recovery. Talk to the midwife and the nurses in the intensive care nursery about your desire to breastfeed. They will assist and support you in fulfilling it.

Start to express as soon as you are able to after the delivery, and express at regular intervals. (See pages 138–9 for directions on expressing.) Do not be distressed if you can express only small amounts of milk. Looking at a picture of your baby while you express may stimulate your let-down reflex. Your partner or a friend could investigate for you the possibility of hiring an electric breast pump; many women who are expressing for prolonged periods find these pumps less tiring than hand expression. Expressing by hand at the beginning and end of each session will increase the level of nipple stimulation.

If your baby is not taking the milk, it can be frozen and offered to her at another time. (See page 139 for freezing and storing instructions.)

Talk to other parents with sick or premature babies. There are support groups that offer advice and inexpensive rental of equipment. (See page 243 for contact numbers and addresses.)

Once your baby has started to breastfeed, your milk supply will improve with the extra stimulation provided by suckling. It may assist in building up your milk supply if you finish each breastfeed by hand expressing for five minutes, until your baby is sucking strongly.

Breastfeeding and the working woman

For many years, women felt it was impossible to combine breastfeeding with paid employment, and weaned their babies as a matter of course when they returned to work. Attitudes have changed, and many women now successfully combine work and full or partial breastfeeding.

There are many benefits in continuing breastfeeding, the main one being that it ensures that you have a quiet time of close contact with your baby, several times a day. It is advisable to be at home with your baby for the first six weeks, longer if possible. This gives you time for your lactation to become established. After four months, solids can be introduced into the baby's diet, so there is less need for breastmilk. It may be worthwhile establishing a more ordered pattern of feeding before returning to work.

Several different combinations of feeding patterns can be used, from fully breastfeeding (if you can arrange to be with your baby at all feeding times) to giving your baby a bottle of formula when you are not available. The usual feeding pattern is to breastfeed when you are at home and offer expressed breastmilk or formula at other times. You may find it reassuring to start offering a small amount of breastmilk in a bottle each day about six weeks before you plan to return to work. Do this prior to a feed; 20 mL ($2/3$ fl oz) is plenty.

Many women find expressing difficult and time-consuming, but for your own comfort, and for the maintenance of an adequate supply of breastmilk, it may be necessary. As your baby's need for frequent feeds gradually lessens and solids form a greater part of her diet, the need for you to express will be reduced.

If you are expressing breastmilk at work, it may help if you take a picture of your baby to work and look at the picture when you are expressing your milk, to assist in the letting-down process. Negotiate with your employer a quiet, private area that you can use while you express. If the door will not lock, make a 'Do not disturb' sign to put on the door to ensure privacy. Remember to store the expressed breastmilk in the central, back part of the refrigerator (label the bottle or put it in a paper bag with your name on it), and take a cold carry pack in which to transport the expressed breastmilk home.

Expressing breastmilk

To express breastmilk for storage, you will need a **sterile plastic container** for the milk (see pages 164–5) for sterilisation instructions), a **breast pump**, if you are using one, and a **towel** to protect your clothing. Wash your hands before you begin.

Before expressing, try to relax, as this will make expressing easier. Expressing straight after a feed is usually found to be successful by many mothers. If this is not possible and you are at home, you may find having a warm shower, with the water running onto your back, relaxing. If you find expressing painful or difficult, doing it under the shower may help, though you will have to discard this milk, as it will be difficult to keep sterile. The use of warm washers (not too hot; always test on your inner arm before applying to the breast) placed on your breast just before you start to express may also help. Do not be disappointed if you are unable to express large amounts of milk. Planning is the secret to success; if you are wanting enough milk to replace a feed so you can go out, start expressing at least three days before you need the milk.

Massage any lumps prior to expressing. A general massage of the breast is a good idea, as it will encourage the letting down of your milk. Sit in a comfortable position and support your breast with one hand. Gently massage your breasts with the flats of your fingers, using a circular motion, commencing above the breast. Slowly and gently move around the entire breast, always massaging in towards the nipple. This should be done several times to ensure that the whole breast is massaged. You may prefer to do this under a warm shower. Gently stimulate your nipples by drawing them out or rolling them between your fingers.

To **hand express**, hold your breast at the outer edges of the areola (where the pigmented area meets the breast), press your fingers and thumbs together rhythmically, moving them around the areola so as to empty all the ducts. The container you use to collect the milk should have a wide mouth; it is very difficult to direct the flow of milk into the narrow neck of a feeding bottle. If your fingers start to tire, change hands, but try to maintain a rhythm similar to the sucking of your baby. Take care not to be too vigorous when hand expressing, as this may damage the soft tissue of your breast.

Many women find using a hand or electric **breast pump** less tiring or messy than hand expression. When using a breast pump, it is important to follow the directions provided by the manufacturer, and to take care not to damage your nipples or breasts by positioning the pump incorrectly or applying excessive suction.

There is a risk of lactation becoming inadequate if for any reason expressing is replacing your baby's breastfeeds. To reduce this risk, it may be helpful to finish expressing your breasts by hand for a few minutes. This gives increased stimulation to the nerve fibres of the nipples and ensures the emptying of all the ducts.

The parts of the breast pump that come in contact with your breastmilk should be sterilised prior to use, to reduce the risk of contaminating the milk (see pages 164–5 for sterilising instructions).

Storage of breastmilk

Great care needs to be taken when storing breastmilk, as contamination of the milk can easily occur. The risk can be reduced if you always use sterile containers and wash your hands carefully.

Breastmilk should always be stored in plastic containers, as there is less risk of its composition altering than if it is stored in glass. Small sterile bags, specifically designed for storing breastmilk, are available from your chemist. If you are storing a day's supply, you can use plastic feeding bottles, in which the milk can be heated and fed directly to your baby.

If you are **freezing** the milk, pour it into a sterile plastic container, labelled with the date and the approximate amount of breastmilk. Only fill the container three-quarters full, as the frozen milk will expand and the container may burst. Make sure you have sealed the container correctly. Cool it first in the refrigerator, then place it in the freezer. Breastmilk should not be frozen for long periods of time as the milk can be contaminated by bacterial growth, and if offered to your baby can cause infection and illness. Some freezers have a defrost cycle, during which the milk may become partly thawed so that bacteria can grow.

Breastmilk can be stored for one week in the freezer of a one-door refrigerator, such as a bar fridge; two weeks in the freezer section of a two-door refrigerator; or three months in a deep freezer or a freezer with a separate temperature control.

Breastmilk should be thawed quickly by placing the container in warm water. Do not thaw it in a microwave, as this will alter its composition. Shake the breastmilk well before offering it to your baby.

When you need help

The best support you can have when breastfeeding is from close family members and friends who have breastfed a baby. Unfortunately, they are not always available and often do not have the specialised skill to help when breastfeeding problems arise. Therefore it is important to find professional support people who understand your needs.

There are two types of support agencies—health professionals and lay trained people or self-help groups. The first support person to locate is your early childhood health nurse, who offers a free service. The nurses on the 24-hour Parent Help Lines or your local doctor can also offer support and reassurance. These health professionals will refer you to parentcraft hospitals or lactation consultants if necessary.

The Nursing Mothers' Association of Australia (NMAA) offers a free telephone counselling service, as well as discussion groups for breastfeeding mothers or those interested in breastfeeding. Other more specific self-help groups may help if your baby has a special problem with breastfeeding—Cleft Pals, for babies with cleft palates, is one such organisation.

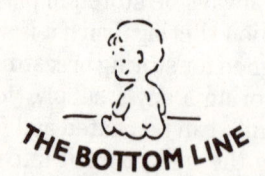

THE BOTTOM LINE

- Your breastmilk is the best food for your new baby.
- Care of your body, especially of your breasts, is an important part of caring for your baby.
- Correct positioning is the key to successful breastfeeding.
- Having a caesarean section, having twins, a premature baby or a sick baby, or returning to work need not prevent you breastfeeding.
- Sterilise anything that is likely to come into contact with expressed breastmilk, and wash your hands before expressing.
- If you need help at any time, don't be embarrassed to ask for it.
- If you need to replace a breastfeed with a bottle, start expressing at least three days before you need the milk.

CHAPTER 11

Common breastfeeding problems

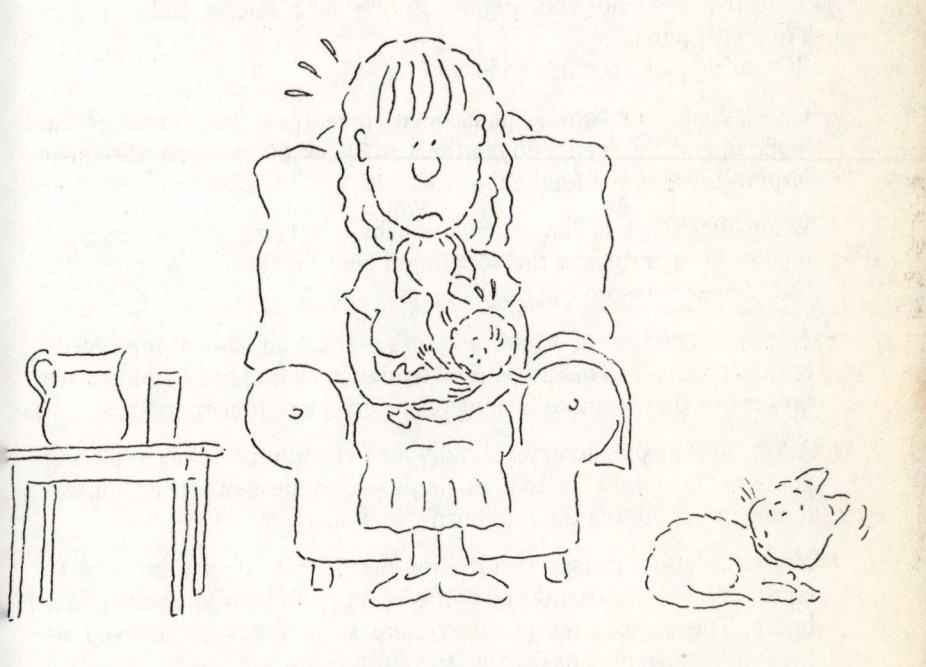

As with most aspects of childcare, breastfeeding does not always progress without a hitch, and it can be unnerving, especially if you are a first-time nursing mother, if things start to go wrong. There are a number of purely physical difficulties you may encounter while you are breastfeeding, and it is best to be aware of them before they happen. This chapter covers the most common of these problems and suggests appropriate action for you to take. If problems arise, seek help from a health professional who has the time to watch you breastfeed, so that she can assess your individual needs.

Tender nipples

A common problem in the first few days for breastfeeding mothers is discomfort associated with sucking due to the new sensation of negative pressure caused by the baby's suck. Tender nipples may also occur during the first few days of breastfeeding. The main cause of tender or cracked nipples is incorrect attachment of your baby to the breast. Other factors that may contribute to your nipple problems are excessive use of creams on your nipples, a thrush infection, breast pads with plastic backing that prevents your nipples drying out properly, and incorrect use of breast pumps.

If your nipples become tender or cracked:

- Check that your baby is positioned correctly at the breast at the beginning of the feed, and continue to check his position at regular intervals during the feed.

- When attaching and detaching your baby, take care not to damage the nipple. Always release the suction on your breast by inserting your little finger between the baby's gums.

- At the completion of a feed, express a small amount of breastmilk onto your nipple. This breastmilk is high in fat and has anti-infective properties that promote healing of any cracks or tender spots.

- Allow your nipples to dry naturally for five minutes before replacing your bra. You might like to use a hairdryer, on the cool setting, for two minutes, but take care not to burn yourself.

- If breastfeeding causes you discomfort or pain, it may be wise to consider hand expressing and bottlefeeding your baby for twenty-four hours. The use of hand or electric breast pumps is not advised, as they may cause further damage to your nipples.

- When having your daily shower, avoid the use of soap on your nipples, as this strips them of their natural oil.

If your nipples remain tender or cracked, seek advice from your early childhood health nurse or lactation consultant. She will check the positioning of your baby and offer suggestions, as well as checking your baby's mouth for signs of **oral thrush**, though it is not always obvious. Thrush infections may be transferred from the baby's mouth to your nipples, and will stop your nipples from healing. Your doctor will recommend an antifungal preparation to clear up the thrush. You should treat your baby's mouth and your nipples at the same time. Remember to wash your hands well before handling your breasts or your baby.

Breast engorgement

Breast engorgement is usually due to an excessive accumulation of milk in the ducts. It is important that you check your breasts for lumps or tender areas after each feed and express if this is necessary to make your breasts comfortable and to remove any lumps, or if a feed is missed. Breast fullness (increased vasularity) commonly occurs during the first few days after you have your baby, when your milk is 'coming in'— this can go on to become engorgement. It can be reduced by putting your baby to the breast for frequent, longer periods. However, this may not be feasible for any number of reasons, including a very sleepy baby, a jaundiced baby, a mother who is anxious or in pain with an episiotomy or caesarean wound, or the presence in the mother's body of drugs given during delivery.

If your breasts are engorged, expressing a small amount of milk to reduce any swelling around the nipple, prior to attaching your baby, will make positioning him easier. A firm, supportive bra and the use of a cool pack (a wet washer wrung out and placed in a plastic bag in the freezer for a short period works well) after expressing will provide some pain relief and help reduce the engorgement. Expressing while in the shower with the warm water running onto your back may relax you and make expressing easier.

Mastitis

Mastitis is the inflammation of the breast; it is usually complicated by an infection. This infection may be due to a blocked duct or an infection spreading into the duct from a cracked nipple.

Engorgement may be one of the first signs of infectious mastitis, but a general feeling of being unwell soon follows, with a raised temperature and extreme tiredness. The breast will be swollen, tender and painful to touch. A reddened area may appear on the surface of the affected breast. Your first response should be to feed your baby and, if necessary, take medication (paracetamol) for pain. The use of cold packs between feeds and a warm pack just prior to feeding is effective. Avoid vigorous massage; gently stroke the breast.

You should consult your doctor as soon as you suspect that you have mastitis, as oral antibiotic treatment may be needed. Remember to complete the course of tablets to prevent the bacteria building up a resistance to the drug. You should start to feel better within forty-eight hours. *It is important to continue breastfeeding your baby*, as this will be less painful than expressing milk. If possible, position your baby so that his chin is pointing in the direction of the reddened area, to allow the emptying of that area of the breast. This may involve feeding him twin fashion (with his body under your arm) or upside down, with his legs lying against your shoulder while you lie down, for part of the feed. Your baby has a most efficient suck that will assist in emptying your breast, although it may be necessary to express after each feed to make your breast feel comfortable. Use the same method of treatment as for engorgement.

If you have a history of mastitis:

- avoid missing feeds or going for prolonged periods without expressing;
- use a variety of feeding positions, to ensure that all milk ducts are emptied;
- if your baby is not emptying your breasts, express a little milk before feeding to encourage him to drain your breasts at the end of the feed;
- examine your breasts for lumps after every feed, and massage or express if necessary to remove the milk in these areas;
- be aware of the fullness of your breasts, and if they are overfull or uncomfortable, feed your baby or express the excess milk; and
- avoid sleeping in a bra.

Flat or inverted nipples

Difficulties attaching your baby to the breast may arise if you have flat or inverted nipples. Time is the most important factor in compensating for these; as your baby becomes more alert and sucks more strongly, and your confidence in handling him grows, it will become easier to attach him to the breast. You can make feeding easier. Express a small amount of milk at the beginning of each feed, using a breast pump; this will help draw out your nipples. Save this milk to offer to your baby at the completion of the feed if necessary.

The use of a nipple shield may be helpful, until your baby can be attached. Always try to attach him without the shield at the beginning of the feed and again during the feed as the nipple will have been drawn out. If the shield is used throughout the feed allow him to feed for longer, as the negative pressure is not as strong through the shield. Express at the end of the feed to give additional stimulation to your breasts; prolonged use of a nipple shield may cause your milk supply to diminish. Nipple shields come in a variety of shapes and materials. Silicone nipple shields are the most efficient and comfortable, as they are thinner and give greater amounts of stimulation. Take care to sterilise them prior to use (see pages 164–5 for sterilisation instructions). If you are unable to cease the use of the shield, you should seek the advice and assistance of your early childhood health nurse or a lactation consultant.

Avoid trying to attach your baby to the breast for prolonged periods, as you and your baby may become frustrated and upset. It is far better to use a nipple shield, and try again to attach your baby to the breast halfway through the feed, when you are both calmer.

Insufficient milk

If your baby is not gaining weight in the first few weeks, or is unsettled, one reason may be that he is not receiving enough milk. Then again, there may be a quite different reason for his behaviour. It is important that you consult your early childhood health nurse for advice, assessment of your baby and your breastfeeding technique and, if necessary, referral to other health professionals, before embarking on a programme to increase your breastmilk supply.

For many women, the problem of insufficient breastmilk can be easily rectified. There are many reasons why your breastmilk supply may be diminishing: not taking enough care of yourself, missing out on much-needed sleep, and high levels of anxiety. Other reasons may be inadequate stimulation of your breasts caused by a sleepy or sick baby, or a reduction of the number of breastfeeds offered.

To increase your breastmilk supply:

- Examine, and if necessary improve, your physical health. Are you getting enough sleep? Is your diet well balanced? Are you taking plenty of fluids? Are you relaxed and exercised?
- Feed your baby more frequently, and for as long as he wishes, for a few days, decreasing the time between feeds. Every two-and-a-half to three hours is usually sufficient. Don't increase feeds to the point where you become exhausted.
- Offer both breasts at each feed, if possible.

- Hand express for five minutes after each feed, to increase breast stimulation. This milk can be stored to feed to your baby later.
- If you need to offer your baby extra fluids, (only 4–6 times per day) always do so after the breastfeed. A lact-aid (a container with a fine tube that you can connect to the side of your nipple) may be used, which still allows your baby to suck on the breast, thus providing necessary breast stimulation.
- Try to relax before you commence each breastfeed, as this will improve the letting down of your milk.
- Maintain your confidence in your ability to breastfeed. This may involve reading books and pamphlets about breastfeeding, or talking to a breastfeeding counsellor or another nursing mother.

Fast flow

A fast flow of breastmilk usually occurs at the beginning of a feed when you let down, or during the feed if you have more than one let down. You may find that your baby chokes and splutters, or even detaches himself from the breast, when the flow of milk is too fast. A fast flow is not necessarily an indication of an abundant milk supply, but should be assessed by your early childhood health nurse or a lactation consultant.

If a fast flow is a problem, it may help to express for a few minutes prior to the commencement of the feed; this will assist in taking the initial gush of milk away and help him attach more easily. Also check that you have positioned your baby correctly (see page 132). Learn to interpret your baby's behaviour and his sucking at the breast. It may be necessary to change your position as his sucking changes. This is usually a temporary problem, that normally resolves itself by six weeks. The early childhood health nurse may be a valuable support person during this time, assessing the way you are feeding and providing practical advice and assistance.

Oversupply

Oversupply is a problem for many women, particularly in Australia for some reason. The breasts work on supply and demand and frequently in the early stages they are prepared to feed more than one baby. This problem can take up to six weeks to settle down.

Signs of oversupply are an unsettled infant who possets frequently and has explosive bowel motions. In many cases there is an associated fast flow. One way to manage oversupply is to offer one breast at a time and let the baby completely empty it. The baby may be reluctant to suck once the flow has slowed so it is important to re-offer the first breast until it is empty. Another way is to express before feeding. Unlike expressing after a feed, expressing prior to a feed will not increase the milk supply. This will enable the baby to feed more comfortably and reach the hind-milk which is higher in fat. The amount that is necessary to express will vary, and it should be gradually reduced over a period of time until the supply equals the baby's demands. The early childhood health nurse or lactation consultant will help with a regime.

Leaking breastmilk

The problem of leaking breastmilk commonly occurs during the early days of breastfeeding, before your milk supply has had a chance to settle into a pattern of supply and demand. It can continue if your muscle control is poor.

To cope with leaking breastmilk, wear a bra that provides even support. Use breast pads inside it to soak up any excess milk. You can buy disposable or washable breast pads from chemists or supermarkets, or simply use a face washer folded into four. Change pads regularly, as they can be a great source of infection, especially if you have tender nipples. Do not use plastic-backed pads, as they will increase the risk of infection by increasing the temperature of the leaked milk. When you have any sensation of leaking, apply pressure to your nipple with the palm of your hand, or your forearm. When feeding, it may be helpful if you allow the second breast to drip while your baby feeds from the first; it may be getting rid of extra breastmilk, and will make feeding from the second breast easier for the baby by taking away any initial gush of milk.

Wearing patterned colourful outfits may help disguise the wet spots on your clothing.

Breast refusal

Your baby may refuse the breast for one of any number of reasons: the commencement of your menstruation, ovulation, a second pregnancy, a low milk supply or a fast flow of milk, or your baby having a blocked nose from a cold. You may be able to identify the cause of his refusal, or you may not. In most cases it is only a transient problem that will resolve itself, given enough time.

FEEDING YOUR BABY

To cope with breast refusal:

- Don't allow your baby to become too hungry before offering him the breast. Try offering the breast when your baby is just starting to stir.

- Find a quiet place to feed, and try to relax before beginning to feed.

- Having another person available to calm your baby down if he becomes distressed may be helpful.

- Express milk at the beginning of a feed to stimulate your let-down reflex in readiness for the baby.

- Check that your baby is not unwell and can breathe freely through his nose. You may need to reposition him on the breast so that he can breathe. Try placing him on the breast twin fashion.

- With an older baby, you may be offering too large a quantity of solids for him to need any breastmilk; offer the breastfeed before the solids. Consider the possibility that your baby may simply not need as many breastfeeds as previously. Take into account your baby's age; around six months babies are easily distracted.

- Try expressing your breastmilk (see pages 137–8 for techniques) and offering it in a bottle for a few feeds, to appease your baby's hunger without involving you both in a battle to put him to the breast. (Give your baby extra cuddles, and yourself plenty of care and attention, to compensate for the absence of the closeness you both obtain from breastfeeding.) Re-offer the breast when you are both calm and relaxed.

- If your milk supply is low, try the methods suggested on page 145.

- Remain calm; never force your baby onto your breast.

It can be worrying and confusing when your baby refuses the breast, but such problems are quick to resolve, given time and patience. Stay calm and persist in your efforts to feed your baby naturally. Don't take breast refusal personally; your baby is not rejecting you and the problem is not a reflection on your ability to mother.

It's important to maintain your confidence in your ability to breastfeed if you are encountering difficulties. Do this by talking to other committed breastfeeding mothers or breastfeeding counsellors.

COMMON BREASTFEEDING PROBLEMS

Biting

Being bitten by a breastfeeding baby is a common occurrence. It is usually a surprise, and it can be very painful.

There are many reasons why babies bite the breast. It can occur by accident, or as part of a normal developmental stage (learning to chew). It is a natural reaction to the painful gums that develop with teething. It produces a great reaction from Mum, which many babies find entertaining enough to try to produce again. And sometimes the milk supply diminishes during feeding, and the baby starts to bite instead of suck—it may be worthwhile trying some of the techniques suggested on page 145–6 to increase your milk supply.

Whatever the cause, it is important to minimise your reaction to the bite if possible. Take your baby off the breast and in a flat tone say 'No'. Put him back on the breast. If he bites again, remove him, and do not re-offer the breast for a short period, or even until the next breastfeed is due. Make sure that your breasts are comfortable, and if necessary express for comfort.

An unsettled baby

One of the first pieces of advice you will probably receive if your baby is unsettled is to wean him onto a bottle. There is absolutely no guarantee that your baby will settle once a bottle is offered. In many cases his behaviour is unrelated to the method you are using to feed him; in which cases weaning will make no difference at all.

First, try the usual methods of settling your baby (see pages 69–70). Check the positioning of your baby at the breast (see page 132–3 for a checklist), and make sure that you allow him to finish feeding from the first breast before changing to the other breast (to obtain hindmilk). Follow the suggestions for increasing your milk-supply if you think this is necessary—see page 145–6.

If you yourself are unsettled or stressed, you may be communicating this to your baby. Give yourself some time out and don't punish yourself with accusations of failure. Read chapter 3 on survival techniques; follow the suggestions for keeping your spirits up.

Check that your baby is well. Talk to your early childhood health nurse, who may offer advice and support that help you identify the cause of your baby's unsettled behaviour.

If you think your baby is hungry, seek the help of a professional to assess whether the baby needs additional fluid in the form of cooled

FEEDING YOUR BABY

boiled water, expressed breastmilk or formula—this is not advised before six weeks of age. It is rare for a baby to need extra fluid at all feeds. Give him no more than 60 mL (2 fl oz) at the afternoon and evening feeds. This can be lessened to suit his demands.

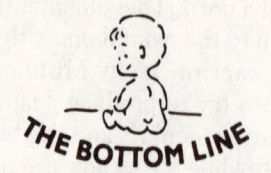

THE BOTTOM LINE

- Your physical and emotional well-being, not only your baby's, is of the first importance when you are breastfeeding.
- Be positive in maintaining your confidence in your ability to breastfeed. Keep in mind clear reasons why you are doing it.
- Always check that your baby is correctly positioned at the breast.
- Allow him to complete feeding at one breast before changing to the second breast.
- Become familiar with the state of your breasts and check them

CHAPTER 12

Weaning

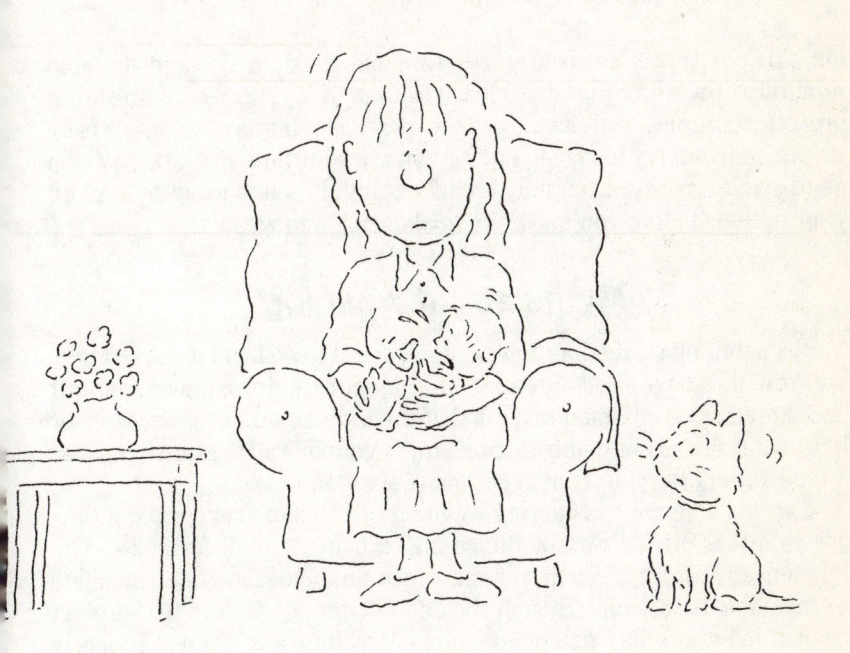

A great deal has been written about breastfeeding but very little information is available about weaning. In many cases weaning occurs naturally, without any fuss or bother, at some time during infancy or toddlerhood.

There are many reasons why you may choose to wean your baby. The important thing is that you feel in control of the decision to wean and the weaning process.

The decision to wean usually occurs after a great deal of discussion and soul-searching about the advantages and disadvantages of breastfeeding versus bottlefeeding. Before starting to wean your baby, it is important that you understand that:

- breastmilk is the ideal milk for most babies during the first twelve months of their lives, but only if breastfeeding is making you and your baby happy;
- it can be very difficult to reverse the decision to wean once you have started to wean, or once your baby is fully weaned; and
- weaning may not be the answer to the problem of an unsettled baby.

On the positive side, remember that babies do grow and develop normally on humanised milk formulas. A system of combining breastfeeding and bottlefeeding can work well for both you and your baby if your milk supply is inadequate, if you are returning to work or if you need some time out from fully breastfeeding. It is important to explore your options before you make the final decision to wean.

Myths about weaning

Myths about infant feeding and weaning seem to go hand in hand. Many women have weaned because of inaccurate information about breastfeeding. A common myth is that the mother's milk is too weak for her infant; this is quite untrue; breastmilk contains all the nutrients that are necessary for your baby until she is six months old.

Parents who are considering weaning can become concerned if they are told that infants do not thrive on humanised milk formulas. The humanised milk formulas that are now recommended have been modified to resemble breastmilk, though they do not contain factors that protect against infection. The risk of infection is low if care is taken to properly sterilise equipment and prepare the formula correctly.

It is not true that when your baby grows teeth you must stop breastfeeding. Many mothers successfully breastfeed babies who have a whole mouthful of teeth.

It is possible to return to work and continue to breastfeed successfully. Returning to work is not a reason to wean, unless you choose to for some other reason.

When to wean

A common question parents ask is 'When do we wean our baby?' There is no right or wrong time to wean your baby. You should breastfeed for as long as you feel happy doing so.

Weaning is not advised, however, when your baby is between

seven and ten months of age, as this is when she reaches a 'peak of attachment'. One of the main characteristics of this period is clinging behaviour due to an apparent need for security.

It is not a good idea to wean when a major crisis or upheaval is occurring in your family. If it is not possible for you to continue breastfeeding as a result, lots of cuddles with your baby will make both of you feel happier and more secure.

Methods of weaning

There are many ways to wean your baby. The method you choose can be adjusted to suit you and your baby.

Gradual weaning involves the phasing in of alternative methods of feeding. The change-over period may be several days or many months. When deciding the time you will take, consider the age of your baby, which will usually determine how many breastfeeds you are offering her. If she is already taking solids, she will be used to other taste sensations and may not be as difficult to wean.

Remember that her behaviour may change during weaning. She may be indifferent to the breast, clinging, refuse to drink from a cup or only take small amounts of fluid from a cup.

The reason you are weaning will largely determine the amount of time you have at your disposal to wean. Must you have your baby weaned by a certain time, or can you take as long as you wish? You may be weaning for medical reasons, in which case there may be a time specified for you to have completed weaning.

A form of gradual weaning is **mutual weaning**; this usually occurs in late infancy or toddlerhood, and involves both you and your baby deciding that it is time to wean. Your milk supply diminishes naturally due to the erratic feeding pattern of your baby, and the function of the breastmilk changes from fulfilling a nutritional need to fulfilling an emotional need (comfort feeding).

Some babies may choose to wean themselves suddenly. This call be distressing and suggestions for dealing with breast refusal (pages 147–8) may assist.

Abrupt weaning is when you make a decision not to breastfeed again. Your baby will go from being fully breastfed to being weaned—there is no change-over period. We *do not recommend* this method of weaning, and it is only used in special circumstances: if your doctor has advised against continuing with breastfeeding because you need to be hospitalised or because of medications you are taking, or if your baby is

FEEDING YOUR BABY

GRADUAL WEANING

- Decide on the time you will take to wean—a week? a month? three months?
- Eliminate feeds that are the least important to you first—perhaps the mid-morning feed could go, or an afternoon feed. Most women maintain the early morning feed, as this is the time of greatest milk supply, and/or the late evening feed, as they can use this feed to settle their baby for the night.
- A possible pattern of elimination could be as follows:

Five feeds over a four-week period

	6 am	10am	2 pm	6 pm	10 pm
weeks 1	breast	bottle	breast	breast	breast
2	breast	bottle	breast	bottle	breast
3	breast	bottle	bottle	bottle	breast
4	breast	bottle	bottle	bottle	bottle

then all bottle feeds

If more than five feeds per day are offered, you can increase the time you will take to wean.

Four feeds over a two-week period

	7 am	12 noon	4 pm	8 pm
days 1	breast	breast	bottle	breast
6	breast	bottle	breast	bottle
10	breast	bottle	bottle	bottle
14	bottle	bottle	bottle	bottle

These patterns should be adapted to fit your way of life, your current feeding pattern and your physical and emotional needs. Remember that there is no right or wrong system when weaning your baby.

refusing the bottle to such an extent that weaning is necessary.

It is important, when abruptly weaning, that you have someone on hand to support you through the weaning period, as it can be a time of high anxiety for both you and your baby. A support person can help by offering the bottle to your baby, which will make feeding easier than if you offer the bottle, when the smell of your breastmilk may distract the baby. Friday evening can be a good time to start weaning, as you often have someone there to support you throughout the weekend.

Warn your neighbours that your baby may cry more than usual, if the crying is likely to disturb them. They may choose to go away for the weekend or, better still, offer you some assistance!

Give your baby lots of physical contact; partners and support people can be of great assistance, providing your baby with cuddles or managing the household while you rest and play with your baby.

Keep a check on your baby's wet nappies; this is a good indicator of your baby's fluid needs. She should produce about the same number of wet nappies as usual. (See page 212 on dehydration.)

Contact your early childhood health nurse, your local doctor or a centre such as Tresillian if you become concerned about your baby's fluid intake or behaviour during the weaning period.

Finally, pay close attention to the condition of your breasts.

The effect of weaning on the mother

There are many physical changes that occur when you wean. Your **breast shape and size** will change, and you may experience an increase or a decrease in your **energy levels** and **weight**.

The **risk of your becoming pregnant** will increase as your hormone levels rise. It may be a good idea to discuss your contraceptive needs with your doctor and your partner. An increase in the frequency of menstruation and the amount of blood flow during menstruation may also occur, so be prepared.

Suppression of lactation means stopping the production of your breastmilk. The use of drugs to suppress lactation is not necessary, if you give yourself adequate time to reduce your milk supply. Suppression of lactation is an individual process that varies in length from woman to woman. It may still be possible to express small amounts of milk from your breasts many months after you have fully weaned your baby.

Excessive milk supply and breast problems should not be a worry if you are mutually weaning, and if you practise the skills of **breast expression and massage** at regular intervals, your milk supply will be suppressed without breast engorgement occurring. Check your breasts and express if necessary at each of your usual feeding times. Express only to make your breasts comfortable, not to empty them of milk; this will not encourage excessive milk production, as expressing is not a good substitute for your baby sucking at the breast.

Wear **a firm, supportive bra** during the weaning period, for your own comfort. Take care not to cause injury to your breasts when you are expressing or massaging them. Massage and express in the shower if you are experiencing problems with your breasts. Allow the water to fall onto your back, as this will relax you and encourage a letting down of your breastmilk.

Warm washers or hand towels applied to your breast just before expressing also aid in the expression of breastmilk. Always test the temperature of the cloth, by holding it against your inner arm for a few seconds. If your breasts are engorged, apply a cold washer or hand towel after feeding or expressing, to reduce swelling.

The habit of breast examination should be a regular ritual for all women, to detect the early occurrence of any breast problems. **Check your breasts** for tender, lumpy or reddened areas, and pay special attention to those areas when massaging and expressing milk from your breasts. Gradually increase the intervals between expression.

If you start to feel unwell or develop a temperature, or if your breasts become tender, seek medical advice. (See pages 143–4 for information on mastitis.)

Emotional changes may occur as your relationship with your baby changes. Many women experience mixed feelings about weaning their babies. These feelings vary from regret and grief to feelings of accomplishment and satisfaction.

During this time of change, it is important to share your feelings with someone sympathetic and to congratulate yourself on having given your baby a good start.

The effect of weaning on your baby

Your baby may also experience a combination of physical and emotional changes. There is a risk of her developing **allergies** as a result of the introduction of a foreign protein. A change in the consistency, colour and odour of her bowel motions is to be expected. She may become unsettled or more settled on the new milk formula: this can be due to an increase or decrease in her fluid intake. Her weight may increase rapidly, or weight gains may slow down.

The **emotional reaction** of your baby will be dependent on her age and the reason you are weaning her. Many babies go through the weaning process without any difficulties and settle quickly onto the humanised milk formula that is offered.

If your baby refuses a bottle

Babies under the age of nine months are generally offered a bottle from which to take their milk. This can be important in continuing the physical closeness parents have with their baby at feeding time and the satisfaction of sucking for the baby. Larger quantities of milk are usually taken by the baby from a bottle than from a cup.

Some babies will refuse a bottle *and* a cup. This can make the weaning process extremely difficult for the parents and the baby. Reasons for refusal include: the baby never having been given a bottle, or having only limited experience in drinking from a bottle; the baby associating a bottle with an unpleasant experience, such as having been force-fed at some stage: or the baby's distress at the sudden separation from her mother.

Expert advice, assistance and support may be necessary. The specialised skill of the early childhood health nurse in infant feeding problems may be useful to you. A close watch on your baby's fluid intake and urinary output is important so that you know when to take measures to prevent your baby becoming dehydrated.

If your baby is refusing to take milk from a bottle and you are unable to continue to breastfeed, the following points may be worth remembering:

- Be gentle and calm in your approach—never force-feed your baby.

- Your partner or a friend may have more success at bottlefeeding your baby at first, as the baby will not smell your breastmilk.

- If the person who is going to feed your baby is unfamiliar with her, encourage them to have a short play period before offering the bottle. This will be less frightening for your baby.

- It is usually the bottle and teat, not what is in the bottle, that causes the baby to refuse the bottle, but you may find that your baby accepts expressed breastmilk more readily in the initial stages of weaning.

- Use an old teat, as its softened condition may be more appealing to your baby. But make sure the teat is in good condition. A new rubber teat boiled for half an hour will become softer.

FEEDING YOUR BABY

- Do not try for prolonged periods to feed your baby. Leave two to four hours between feeds. You and your baby are less likely to become frustrated. Use fresh breastmilk or formula each time, as milk is easily contaminated.

- It is important to give your baby extra cuddles after each attempt to feed.

- During this often difficult period, it is important to have someone to confide in, to help reduce any anxiety or sadness you may be feeling.

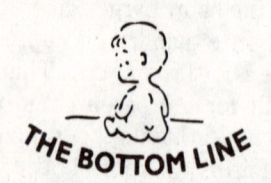

THE BOTTOM LINE

- The decision to wean should be your own, and should be based on factual information and you and your baby's physical and emotional needs.
- Don't feel guilty about your decision to wean your baby; breastfeeding is not the only way to be a 'good mother'.
- Gradual weaning is easier on both parents and baby; if you have to abruptly wean, have lots of physical contact with your baby to compensate for the loss of the closeness of breastfeeding.
- Never force-feed your baby.
- Organise support for yourself during the weaning period.

CHAPTER 13

Bottlefeeding

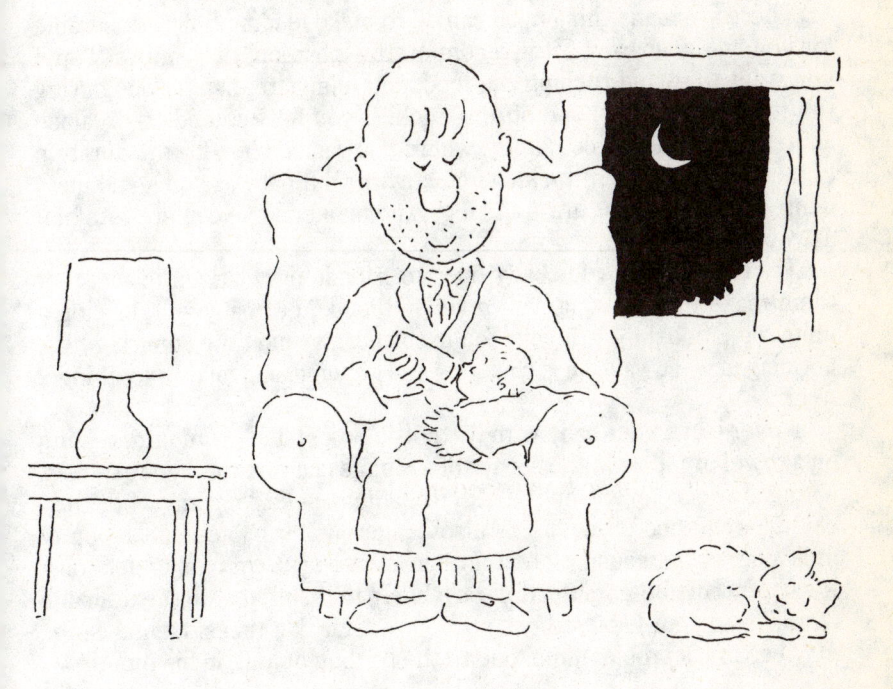

Many women would love to fully breastfeed their babies, but for many different reasons are not able to do so. Bottlefeeding remains an acceptable alternative method of feeding for many parents. Bottlefed babies thrive and grow into well-developed, happy individuals, just as breastfed babies do.

Some breastfeeding women offer the occasional bottle of expressed breastmilk or formula so that they can take some well-earned time out. This can give their partners a chance to feed and get to know the baby, which can be a great confidence booster for new fathers.

Enjoying bottlefeeding

Bottlefeeding can be a time of joy, love and closeness for baby and parents. It is important not to feel guilty about your decision to bottlefeed, regardless of the reason. The bond between baby and parents is dependent on many things, not just the method of feeding.

There are many things you can do to make feeding time pleasurable for you and your baby. Sit in a comfortable position; put your feet up if you want to. Avoid rushing the feed, and eliminate distractions during the feed—take the phone off the hook. If you have a toddler, organise something for her to do quietly, where you can see her, for the duration of the feed. Have skin-to-skin contact with your baby as you feed him—gently stroke his face, arms and legs, and maintain eye contact with him as you feed.

Try not to hand your baby over to friends or relatives to feed; let them make the tea while you relax and feed. Your baby will develop a unique relationship with you. You in turn can spend time admiring him, noticing in what ways he is changing and growing, and talking soothingly to him.

Never leave your baby with the bottle propped in his mouth, resting on a towel or pillow in the corner of a lounge chair or cot. In our society, eating is a social event, and babies, like adults, need company when they eat. This method of feeding is also dangerous for babies. Inhalation of milk may occur, causing breathing problems or respiratory infections. Recurrent middle-ear infections are likely to result, due to the drainage of milk into your baby's short, straight Eustachian tubes. Dental caries may become a problem, too, due to the pooling of milk in his mouth.

Humanised formulas

The milk formulas that have been developed for babies under twelve months of age are called 'humanised' formulas. It is impossible to manufacture a substance that is exactly the same as breastmilk, which is a complex living fluid, but humanised milks resemble it, with the major components in similar proportions. They have a cow's milk base and are a complete food; additional vitamins or iron are not needed, as they are present in the formula in amounts to suit most babies' needs.

Humanised milks are recommended, in preference to cow's or goat's milk, during the first nine to twelve months of your baby's life. There is too much salt in cow's and goat's milk for your baby's immature kidneys to cope with, as well as protein curds that are difficult to digest and pose a high risk of allergy. Also, lactose (sugar of milk) and vitamins are not present in them in sufficient amounts once they have been diluted for the baby's feed.

There are two groups of humanised milk: whey-based and casein-based. Both are produced using cow's milk. In **whey-based** milks the protein curd is lighter and easier to digest. These are recommended for babies under six months of age, but can be given to babies over six months. It is not necessary to change from a whey-based formula after six months if your baby is content with this formula. In **casein-based** milks the protein curd is heavier and takes a greater effort to digest. These milks are recommended for babies over six months of age.

Soya milk formulas

Formulas based on soya milk, obtained from soya beans, are an alternative to humanised milks. These formulas provide sucrose (cane sugar) as the main energy source instead of the lactose in cow's milk-based formulas.

Some reasons why parents choose soya-based milks are:

- Parents choose to avoid animal products in their diets.

- About 1–3 per cent of babies have an intolerance to cow's milk, and some of these babies are able to tolerate soya milk.

- Babies who are unable to tolerate lactose are usually able to tolerate soya milk.

If you choose to use a soya milk formula, use only formulas that have been fortified to meet the nutritional requirements of a baby, including added calcium. These formulas are prepared using the same method as humanised formulas. If you need further advice about the use of soya milk formulas, talk to your early childhood health nurse or local doctor.

Preparing formula

Most milk formulas come in a **powdered** form. Always wash your hands before preparing the powder, and set up your sterilised equipment (see pages 164–5). Avoid distractions when preparing the formula, so that you can be sure you have made it up correctly. Take the phone off the hook, and keep pen and paper handy so that you can make a note of where you are up to if you are interrupted.

FEEDING YOUR BABY

There are two recommended methods of preparing the powder:
1. (a) Measure the cooled boiled water into a measuring jug with clear levels marked on the side.
   (b) Using the scoop from the formula tin, measure the required number of scoops into the measuring jug. Use a knife to level off each scoop.
   (c) Whisk the mixture to dissolve the powder.
   (d) Store the mixture in the centre back of the refrigerator in either the covered jug or individual feeding bottles.

2. (a) Measure the amount of cooled boiled water required into individual bottles.
   (b) Using the scoop from the formula tin, measure the required number of scoops into the bottles. Use a knife to level off each scoop.
   (c) Cap the bottles and shake each one until the powder has dissolved into the water.
   (d) Store the bottles in the centre back of the refrigerator.

If you are using a **liquid** formula:

- Scald the top of the formula tin by pouring boiling water over it.
- Measure the amount of formula required into a jug or bottle.
- Add the required amount of cooled boiled water.
- Whisk or shake to mix.
- Cap the bottle or jug and store it in the refrigerator.
- The opened tin can be stored in the refrigerator for twenty-four hours, covered with plastic cling wrap.

All types of milk should be stored carefully. Milk is an ideal environment for bacteria to thrive in. Contaminated milk is dangerous for your baby, causing diseases such as gastroenteritis (infection of the gut). Store prepared formula in the centre back of the refrigerator, not in the door. Discard any unused formula after twenty-four hours.

Precautions

- Always wash your hands before preparing formula.
- Use equipment that has been sterilised (see pages 164–5 for directions).

BOTTLEFEEDING

- Use only water that has been boiled for five minutes and then cooled to make up formula; this prevents the heat destroying vitamins in the formula.
- Mix powder and water well.
- Use powder or liquid strictly as directed on the tin.
- Don't add extra scoops of powder to the mixture, as this may cause your baby to become irritable, constipated or dehydrated.
- Store tins of powdered formula in a cool, dry cupboard.
- Make sure you check the expiry date on each tin, and discard it if it is out of date.
- Discard any opened tin of powder after one month.

Heating formula

Heat formula just prior to a feed. Place the feeding bottle in a container of hot water for approximately five minutes, while you are changing your baby's nappy or having a cuddle.

Take care when heating the formula. Keep your baby away from the container, so that you don't burn yourself or him with the hot water. Avoid carrying your baby and the container of hot water at the same time.

Always shake the formula gently before testing its temperature, so that the heat is well distributed through it. Always test the formula on the inner part of your forearm.

The use of a microwave to heat the bottle is not recommended because of the potential for overheating the milk and causing burns to your child's mouth. It also destroys vitamins in the milk.

You will need to discard any leftover milk after each feed; **do not reheat and use it.**

Transportation of formula

When transporting milk, be sure to keep it chilled. Never transport it when it is warm, as this encourages the growth of bacteria in it. It is safer to transport the cool boiled water and the powdered formula in separate containers, eliminating the need to keep the milk always at a constant temperature. They can be mixed together whenever you need formula.

FEEDING YOUR BABY

Bottles and teats

There are many types of bottles and teats on the market. Some manufacturers make amazing claims about the properties of the bottles and teats they produce. Keep in mind that cost does not always reflect the quality of a product.

There are a number of basic qualities you should look for. **Bottles** should be easy to clean (avoid bottles with numerous removable parts, novelty bottles or abnormally shaped bottles), and unbreakable (made of heat-resistant plastic or glass).

The number of bottles you will need is dependent on the number of bottlefeeds your baby has daily, your financial state and your personal preference. We would suggest a minimum of three bottles.

Teats should be of the same brand as the bottles and for a better fit should be made of silicone or rubber; have a slow to medium flow (about one drop per second — with wide-necked bottles this flow can be controlled slightly by loosening or tightening the screw cap); and be good and sturdy, if your baby has a tendency to chew.

You should buy a minimum of three teats. If you keep these constantly sterilised, you will always have a back-up if you happen to drop one on the floor when preparing to feed your baby. Also, if you rotate the use of the teats, it is easier to phase in a new teat when necessary. Some babies will refuse a new teat if they are used to using only one.

Always throw out bottles that are chipped or cracked and teats that are starting to perish.

Cleaning and sterilisation

All equipment that comes into contact with the milk formula should be sterilised until your baby is twelve months old.

To clean **bottles**:

- Rinse them with cold water as soon as the feed is finished.
- Wash them in warm water and detergent.
- Use a bottle brush to remove milk curd and to reach all parts of the bottle. Pay special attention to any ridges or uneven surfaces.

To clean **teats**:

- Rinse them in running water.
- Gently rub the surfaces of the teat together.

- Squeeze warm water and detergent through the teat.
- Turn the teat inside out and rub away any milk curd caught on the edge of the hole.

Chemical sterilisation

Chemical sterilisation is the sterilisation method preferred by Tresillian, as it is more efficient and the potential for accidents is less than that involved in sterilisation by boiling. An anti-bacterial solution is mixed with cold water, and bottles, teats and dummies are placed in the solution. This method takes a minimum of one hour. Anti-bacterial tablets mixed with water will also take a minimum of an hour to sterilise equipment adequately. It is important to follow the manufacturer's instructions. Equipment can be left in the anti-bacterial solution for an unrestricted time, as long as the solution is changed every twenty-four hours.

For chemical sterilisation you will need:

- **Anti-bacterial solution or tablets.** There are several brands on the market. If you are in doubt as to which is best, discuss the matter with your early childhood health nurse or your chemist.
- **A large covered container,** with an inside plate that has numerous holes in it. This will assist in the submersion of all equipment. The holes will allow any air pockets or bubbles to be eliminated. These containers are commercially available.
- **An accurate measuring cup or jug,** for making up the solution. This should not be the same one you mix up your formula in or use for measuring food.

Precautions

- Always read the instructions on the packet or container.
- Never place metal objects in the solution; they will quickly corrode.
- Rinse equipment well before placing it in the solution.
- Make sure there are no air bubbles in bottles or equipment, as the surfaces against which these bubbles rest will not be sterilised.
- All equipment should be covered completely by the solution.
- Always leave objects in the solution for the time advised by the manufacturer.

FEEDING YOUR BABY

- Always wash your hands well before putting them into the solution to remove equipment.

- Change the solution every twenty-four hours. Wash out the storage container with soapy, hot water and rinse it well before making up the new solution.

- Store concentrate and solution out of the reach of children.

Sterilisation by boiling

Sterilisation by boiling is another method that can be used.

- Place bottles, teats and equipment to be sterilised in a large saucepan. You may need to sterilise the bottles separately.

- Fill the saucepan with cold water, until all the equipment is covered. Place a lid on the saucepan.

- Bring the water to a rapid boil and boil it for ten minutes. For safety, use the back jets or rings of the stove, and turn the saucepan handle inwards.

- Remove the bottles, teats and equipment with tongs. If you have older children, it is important that they are kept away during this part of the procedure, so that the boiling water is not splashed or tipped on them. It might be best to sterilise equipment after they have gone to bed.

- Store the bottles with their caps or lids on; teats and other equipment should be put in a sealed, sterilised container. Wash your hands before handling sterilised equipment.

- All bottles, teats and equipment should be sterilised after use or, if not used, every twenty-four hours.

Steam sterilisers work in a similar way to old-fashioned pressure cookers. They usually take four to six bottles, and take about five minutes to sterilise them.

How much milk to offer, and when

Your baby's appetite will vary from feed to feed, so avoid being strict with the frequency of feeds. A three- to five-hourly routine works well. Allow your baby to take the amount he wishes from the bottle, and never force him to finish the bottle. If you provide an environment that is calm and conducive to feeding, your baby will drink adequate amounts of formula for his needs. Your early childhood health nurse will help you to understand your baby's needs, or you can read the label on the formula tin or bottle and follow the weight and age guide suggested by the manufacturer.

Your best guide to the amounts needed for your baby is his behaviour. Does he settle after feeds? Does he have frequent wet nappies, at least one per feed, and is his urine pale and without a strong odour? Are his bowel motions soft and regular? Is his weight in proportion with his height and head circumference (you can have this checked by your early childhood health nurse or your doctor)? And is he bright-eyed, with clear skin? If the answer to any of these questions is no, your baby may not be getting enough food.

Feeding your baby

- Place the baby's bottle in a container of hot water to heat it.

- Change your baby if it is necessary, washing your hands afterwards.

- Test the milk by shaking several drops onto the inner part of your forearm. It should feel lukewarm.

- Sit in a comfortable position, and cradle your baby in your preferred arm.

- Gently place the bottle in your baby's mouth. Check that the teat is on top of his tongue. Hold the bottle at an angle that prevents any air passing into the teat. Gently place your index and middle fingers under your baby's chin. This supports the chin and helps ensure an adequate sucking motion. This step is not necessary for older babies. Never force your baby to suck.

- Babies need a minimum of twenty minutes' sucking time to satisfy their sucking urge. A feeding time of between twenty and forty minutes is recommended. Relax and enjoy this time with your baby. Be aware of his sucking pattern. It should remain smooth and rhythmical. All babies pause for short periods during their feed; do not be disturbed by these pauses.

- Most babies need to stop about halfway through the feed to be burped or winded (see page 66 for guidance). Your baby will not always finish his bottle. Discard any milk that is left over.

The working parent and bottlefeeding

The decision to return to work is usually a difficult one to make for most parents. The many practical and emotional issues involved are discussed in chapter 18, 'Leaving your baby in care'. If your baby is breastfed, you may be worried that he will not take a bottle while you are at work. It is worthwhile having practice runs, so that your baby becomes accustomed to taking a bottle from someone else who is familiar before having to take it from a new carer. It's also worthwhile leaving your baby with the carer for short periods to begin with, so that the transition to the new situation is not too sudden.

As regards feeding, you will need to consider the following points:

- Will you make up the formula or will the carer?

- If the carers are preparing the formula, do they know how to prepare it correctly? Are they aware of the importance of hygiene and the sterilisation of equipment?

- How many bottles will be needed while you are away? (It's a good idea to leave extra formula, in case a bottle is spilt or you are running late.)

- How will you transport the formula if your baby is being cared for away from home?

The unsettled bottlefed baby

It is important to seek professional advice and help if your baby is continually unsettled, regardless of the cause, to reassure yourself that illness is not causing your baby's behaviour.

There are many ways to help your baby settle after a feed. Pages 69–70 list some methods to try. If you have tried these and your baby is still restless, some adjustment of your feeding practice may be necessary.

Try using a slower teat; this will increase your baby's sucking time and may improve his sucking pattern. Avoid taking longer than forty minutes, though, or you and your baby will end up frustrated and tired. You could try using a slower teat for the first ten minutes of the feed, when your baby is hungry and tends to gulp. Then change to a faster teat to finish the feed, as he becomes satisfied and his sucking slows.

Check your method of formula preparation. Are you making the formula as directed? If the formula is too strong or weak, your baby can become unsettled. Are you warming the formula before giving it to your baby? Although formula may be given at room temperature, some babies take it better if it is slightly warmed.

Check your baby's fluid requirements by reading the instructions on the tin of formula or asking your early childhood health nurse about them. Are you overfeeding or underfeeding your baby? See page 212 for the telltale signs of dehydration, and talk to your early childhood health nurse.

Finally, allow adequate time to feed and settle your baby. If you rush him, he will be unsettled.

Before changing formulas or assuming that your baby is allergic to cow's milk protein, check the simple things. Changing from one humanised formula to another is of limited or no benefit, as the basic composition of the formulas is similar. Your baby may improve for one or two days, but if the problem is not resolved your baby will again become unsettled.

Cow's milk allergy

An abnormal immunological reaction (allergy) to cow's milk protein may be due to the immaturity of a baby's digestive and immune systems. This allergy occurs in about 1–3 per cent of babies. The reaction can vary; it may be immediate or delayed by up to forty-eight hours after the baby has had the milk. Reactions vary in severity and may include respiratory problems, skin rashes, vomiting, unsettled behaviour, abdominal pains, diarrhoea and flushing of the skin.

If your baby is suffering from any of these symptoms, consult your doctor, who will prescribe the appropriate treatment and milk formula for your baby.

In the majority of babies with allergies, the reactions lessen with time. In most cases, the baby is able to tolerate most foods, including cow's milk, by the age of two or three years.

If your baby is allergic to cow's milk, you will have to avoid giving him cheese, yoghurt and custards made with cow's milk. This can be very inconvenient for the parents of a baby on a family diet, so make sure your baby has been properly diagnosed.

The sleepy bottlefed baby

If you are concerned that your baby is falling asleep too early during his feeds and not gaining adequate amounts from the bottle, check the following points:

FEEDING YOUR BABY

- Are you offering him too much milk?
- If he is on solids, are you offering him too much food for him to want the bottle? You should offer him the bottle before the solids until he is six months old.
- Is the teat too slow?
- Is your baby's sucking pattern rhythmical? If not, try placing your fingers under his chin, to give it gentle support and resistance to the suck.
- Is your baby unwell? You may need to take him to your doctor or early childhood health nurse for his condition to be assessed.

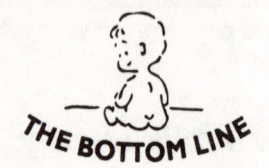

THE BOTTOM LINE

- Take care with the sterilisation of bottles and other equipment used in the preparation of formula.
- Sterilise all such equipment until your baby is twelve months old.
- Offer a humanised formula until your baby is nine to twelve months old.
- Prepare the formula according to the manufacturer's directions. Make sure you measure the formula powder or liquid accurately.
- Store the prepared milk at a constant cold temperature.
- When heating the milk, take care not to overheat it.
- Never force your baby to feed.
- Arrange feeding times so that you can relax and enjoy the time you spend with your baby.

CHAPTER 14

The introduction of solids

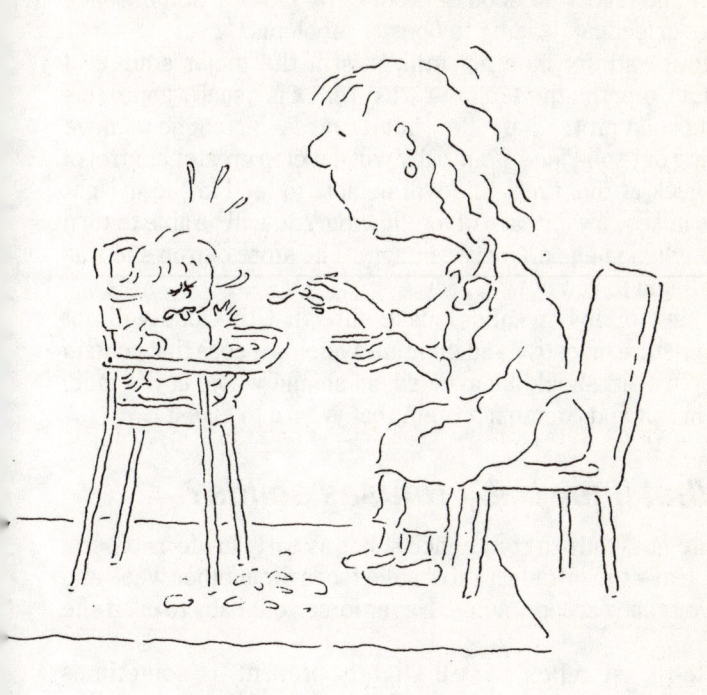

The introduction of solid foods is an important series of events in your baby's life. The growing pleasure she shows in trying new foods and exploring textures and colours is a great reward for parents. One of the most important benefits of feeding your baby solid foods is the interaction that takes place between the baby and yourself at mealtimes.

Many parents take a good look at their own diets when they begin introducing their babies to solid foods. Eating a well-balanced diet yourself is the best way to encourage your baby to eat sensibly. Poor eating habits that become established during babyhood and early childhood can be difficult to change when a child reaches adolescence or adulthood, so now is the time to set firmly in place a family standard of good eating habits.

When should I first offer solid foods?

Babies thrive on breastmilk or humanised formula for the first four to six months of life. There is no need to introduce solids before this time, as it can be time-consuming for parents and difficult for babies if they are not ready to accept and digest the food offered. Early introduction of solids may result in overfeeding, leading to obesity problems.

Between four and six months, milk is still the major source of nutrition. By four months the tongue-thrust reflex is usually gone; this reflex is an important protective reflex, but it causes the tongue to move forward, pushing out solid food. Your baby will develop greater control of her head and neck at this time. She will be able to feed in the upright position that is necessary for ease of swallowing, and will be able to turn her head away when she is no longer hungry. The store of iron she was born with will begin to run out.

When you first offer her solids, make sure that the food will not distress her immature digestive and immune systems. Foods that contain gluten, such as wheat, should be avoided, as should whole cow's milk, which is high in salt and contains protein that is hard to digest.

What if my baby refuses solids?

Some babies are not ready to commence solids as early in life as others. Don't despair; leave the introduction of solid foods for another week and re-offer until your baby accepts some. Never force your baby to eat if she refuses food.

The tongue-thrust reflex, if still slightly present, is sometimes mistakenly interpreted by parents as dislike of the food they are offering their baby, but time and practice in putting food into her mouth is usually all that is needed to encourage your baby to eat.

Seek the advice of your early childhood health nurse if you need assistance in overcoming feeding problems

The type and sequence of solid foods

The best guide to the consistency of food you should be offering your baby is your baby's reaction. Start by offering her food of a consistency like thickened soup. Gradually thicken this to a mashed consistency by about six months.

As your baby grows, and her ability to chew and swallow improves, the consistency of the food you offer her can become more varied. By

A BALANCED DIET

The basis of a well-balanced diet is a varied selection of foods from the following five food groups:

- **Bread, cereals and grains** provide some proteins, minerals, dietary fibre and vitamins. They supply complex carbohydrates, which are important providers of energy.
- **Vegetables and fruit** provide dietary fibre and vitamins. Eat a variety, cooked and raw.
- **Lean meat, fish, poultry, eggs and legumes** (beans, peas and lentils) provide protein, minerals and vitamins. Red meat is an excellent source of iron.
- **Milk, cheese and yoghurt** are excellent sources of calcium, riboflavin, protein, some minerals and vitamins.
- **Butter and table margarine** provide vitamin A (in moderation).

DIETARY GUIDELINES FOR CHILDREN AND ADOLESCENTS

- Try to breastfeed if possible.
- Your child needs appropriate food and physical activity to grow and develop normally. Growth should be checked regularly.
- Offer your child a wide variety of nutritious foods.
- Provide plenty of breads, cereals, vegetables (including legumes) and fruits.
- Low fat diets are not suitable for young children. For older children, a diet low in fat and, in particular, low in saturated fat, is appropriate.
- Encourage water as a drink. Alcohol is not recommended for children.
- Give only a moderate amount of sugars and foods containing added sugars.
- Choose low salt foods.

Guidelines on Specific Nutrients

- Your child needs to eat foods containing calcium.
- Your child needs to eat foods containing iron.

(Adapted from Dietary guidelines for Children and Adolescents NHMRC 1995)

the age of twelve months, she will be able to eat a normal family diet that has been finely chopped or left as finger food.

Introduce chewable foods slowly, so that the development of her facial muscles can occur. This is important for speech development and facial appearance.

The following foods are suggestions only; you may wish to substitute similar foods to suit your family or cultural diet. The important thing is that by twelve months of age, your baby is sharing a well-balanced family diet with foods from the five food groups. It is best to offer fresh food whenever possible. Always offer the breast or bottle first before the age of six months.

Watch for allergic reactions after a new food has been offered to your baby—a common reaction may be unsettled behaviour. *Take your baby to see your local doctor or to the casualty department of your local hospital immediately if a rash appears around her mouth or spots appear on her body; if she has respiratory difficulties, such as wheezing; if any swelling of her lips or throat occurs; if she has diarrhoea or is vomiting; or if she is unsettled and you think she is in pain.*

Rice cereal is the first food that is recommended for babies. It has a low allergy risk and is gluten free, cheap and is iron fortified. The consistency can be varied easily to suit your baby's needs. Start to offer rice cereal when your baby is between four and six months old.

Cereals can be prepared by adding breastmilk, milk formula or cooled boiled water. Start with a teaspoonful and gradually increase to two tablespoons (eight teaspoons). Offer one meal per day, gradually increasing this to two meals per day during the second week.

A variety of mixed cereals can be offered to the older baby of six or seven months. Continue to introduce foods gradually. Nine-month-old babies may enjoy a dessert of creamy rice (rice that has been gently cooked in milk and water until it becomes mushy).

Fruits can be combined with the cereal during the second or third week after commencing rice cereal. This gives your baby a new taste experience and helps prevent constipation. Try one fruit at a time and wait several days to check for allergies before offering another new variety. Apples and pears are usually the safest fruits to start with. Choose ripe fruit, cook it without added sugar, then purée or mash it. Canned fruit can be used if it is processed in its own juice, not a sweetened syrup. The range of fruits you can offer your baby is only limited by the need to wait after introducing each fruit to test for allergic reactions.

Fresh fruit such as very ripe bananas can be mashed with a fork. Stone

THE INTRODUCTION OF SOLIDS

fruits (apricots, peaches, prunes, etc) should be introduced in limited amounts and not more than once a day, because of their laxative effect.

Vegetables can be offered two to four weeks after you begin offering your baby solid foods. Offer a teaspoon of mashed potato first, in the middle of the day, to help start establishing the habit of eating three meals a day. (Many parents find the middle of the day a good time to offer the main meal, as they often have more time and the baby is not as tired.) Stay for several days on this one vegetable before offering another type, such as pumpkin, sweet potato, carrot or parsnip. Avoid mixing the vegetables together until your baby becomes used to the different tastes and textures and you are sure she has no allergic reaction. Gradually introduce other types of vegetables. Frozen vegetables are a good substitute if fresh vegetables are not available.

To prepare fresh vegetables:

- Peel them just before you intend to cook them.

- Don't soak vegetables, as water-soluble vitamins are leached out into the water.

- Steam or microwave the vegetables; cook them until they are soft enough to easily purée, mash or chop, but avoid overcooking.

- Root vegetables such as potato and parsnip can be mashed with a fork.

- Vegetables such as peas and carrots can be blended in a food processor or put through a sieve. Food processors make puréeing and blending baby-sized portions of food very easy.

- Cook extra vegetables when preparing the family meal. They can be stored in a covered container in the refrigerator for your baby's meal the next day.

By six to eight months of age most babies are ready to be offered any type of vegetable, mashed with a fork rather than puréed.

Natural yoghurt can be offered at six to seven months. Start with a teaspoonful and gradually increase. Fresh fruit can be added to make an easy and enjoyable meal for your baby.

Cheeses can be offered, combined with vegetables or fruit. Start with a soft curd cheese, such as ricotta or cottage cheese. Grated cheddar cheese folded through vegetables is a tasty alternative. Your baby will be able to feed herself fingers of cheese. At around twelve months, she will probably enjoy melted cheese on toast as a snack, but take care that the cheese has cooled before offering it to her.

FEEDING YOUR BABY

Meat, chicken and fish can be introduced at around six to seven months. Ensure that these are well cooked to destroy any potentially harmful bacteria. Suitable methods of cooking are steaming, grilling, casseroling or stewing; avoid offering fried foods, as they have a high fat content. The leftover meat from the family meal the night before can be offered to your baby, chopped finely. Red meat is an important source of iron. Make sure that any sauce you serve with the meat does not contain vegetables that have not been tested on your baby for allergy, and that the sauce is not highly seasoned.

Combining the cooking juices with the food you offer, or making a white sauce to go with it, helps moisten the food and provides variety.

At about six or seven months, you can try the following foods:

- cooked flaked fish or chicken mixed with vegetables or finely chopped cooked brains
- grated cheddar cheese on vegetables
- flaked tuna mixed with mashed potato
- milk puddings with well-cooked rice or noodles
- junket and/or mashed banana

Eggs are an important addition to the diet of children. They are a rich source of protein, iron and other minerals, and supply every vitamin except vitamin C. Babies and small children should not be offered raw eggs, as they can carry the salmonella bacteria, which causes gastroenteritis.

At six months, most babies are offered their first taste of egg yolk on a finger of toast. Babies usually enjoy the experience of sucking the egg from the toast. Try this several times, and if your baby does not show signs of allergy, offer her the yolk of a soft-boiled egg.

Egg white can be introduced after eight or nine months, when there is less of a risk of an allergic reaction to the protein in it. Once you know that your baby can tolerate egg, custard can be offered, or any of the following: scrambled egg, savoury egg custard (quiche), hard-boiled egg, or lightly boiled egg mashed with a fork and mixed with breadcrumbs.

From eight months of age, you can offer your baby **finger foods**, but always supervise her, as she can easily choke. Some suggested finger foods are:

- crusts, rusks, fingers of toast with a thin layer of butter or spread (avoid high-salt spreads such as beef or yeast extracts);

- cheese sticks;
- fingers of grilled steak (no gristle or fat);
- quarters of apples or pears, segments of orange;
- lightly steamed vegetables.

Legumes (dried beans, peas and lentils), if prepared correctly, provide a cheap and delicious high protein and iron source for your baby. They should be soaked in water overnight to replace the fluid removed during the drying process. It is also important to boil legumes for a minimum of fifteen minutes before adding them to casseroles or soups for further cooking, as they require prolonged cooking to make them suitable for your baby to eat. Before offering them to your baby, ensure that the legumes can be easily mashed with a fork. Add legumes to casseroles, stews and soups, use them as a substitute for part of the mince in rissoles, or mix them with vegetables and/or cheese.

Foods to avoid

It is not a good idea to offer your baby the following foods:

- fatty foods such as fried meats, the skin of chicken, fish in batter or potato chips;
- raw eggs or undercooked poultry products, as they may contain the salmonella bacteria;
- foods that are very salty or sweet. Avoid adding extra sugar or salt to food that you cook for your child;
- honey, until your child is twelve months old, as it may contain botulism spores;
- nuts or any type of small hard foods—do not give unless crushed until your child is five years old, as there is a high risk of her inhaling the food and choking.

Use commercial spreads for sandwiches in moderation, as they usually have a high salt or oil content.

There is no need to offer lollies or sweet foods such as icecream to very small children. Keep these for a rare and special treat when they are older.

Remember, babies do not have adult palates or tastes, so take care when you are seasoning foods. Foods that taste bland to adults are often enjoyed by babies.

Vegetarian diets

Many parents are choosing to feed their babies a vegetarian diet, as evidence suggests that this is one way to develop healthy eating habits in their children. Tresillian advises parents to seek the advice of a paediatric dietician if they are unsure of the nutritional requirements of their growing baby.

The most frequently used vegetarian diet is the lactovo vegetarian diet, which includes protein-rich foods such as eggs, cheese, milk, grains and legumes, as well as fruits and vegetables. A diet including these foods fulfils all a baby's needs for protein, energy, vitamins and minerals. The lacto-vegetarian diet includes all the above foods except eggs.

Parents who choose to feed their babies on a strictly vegan diet (one that contains no animal products such as cheese, milk or eggs) will need to use supplementary proteins.

If parents choose a vegetarian diet for their baby, it is important that the foods they offer contain adequate amounts of protein, iron, calcium, zinc, riboflavin and vitamin B12, as these nutrients are not always readily available in a vegetarian diet. The foods offered should be in balanced proportions.

Many foods are best offered in combination with others, as they do not contain the eight essential amino acids (proteins). They should be combined with foods containing complementary proteins so that a complete protein is consumed. For example, offer pasta (which contains grain protein) and milk (a milk protein) in macaroni cheese, or beans (a legume protein) and bread (a grain protein) in a baked-bean sandwich.

One of the major problems for babies and small children on vegetarian diets is that they cannot consume enough food for their nutritional needs. Vegetarian diets, if not well designed, tend to be too bulky for a baby's small stomach capacity. If you are unsure about your baby's nutritional needs, discuss them with a dietician who specialises in vegetarian diets. You can find one through the dietician at your local hospital or paediatric hospital.

Fruit juices

If babies are breastfed or offered a humanised or other specialised milk formula until they are six months old, their vitamin requirements are

THE INTRODUCTION OF SOLIDS

SEQUENCE OF SOLID FOODS
(INTRODUCE ONLY ONE FOOD AT A TIME)

4–6 months	rice cereal, fruits and vegetables
6 months	egg yolk, mixed cereals
6 months	meat, chicken and fish
7 months	legumes
8 months	finger foods
9 months	egg white
12 months	whatever the family eats

adequately met during that time. The offering of fruit juice during this period is for its educational value rather than for nutrition, therefore it is not necessary and may cause difficulties if you are still breastfeeding.

The types of juice to offer are freshly squeezed orange, apple or pear juice—all should be diluted before being offered to your baby. Other juices may be offered as your baby grows. Tinned or carton juices are useful for the busy parent, but expensive in the beginning if you are using only a small portion.

Full-strength juice can cause loose bowel motions and burning and reddening of your baby's buttocks. Your baby's teeth can benefit from the fluoride in the water you use to dilute the juice, if your local water supply contains fluoride.

To start your baby on fruit juice, offer her 5 mL (a teaspoonful) of fresh juice to 30 mL (1 fl oz) of cooled boiled water. Each day, increase thie fruit juice by 5 mL, until you are offering her 30 mL of juice to every 30 mL of cooled boiled water. Remember to boil the water for five minutes before leaving it to cool.

If your baby is over seven months of age, juice may be offered in small quantities from a thick-lipped, unbreakable cup or a plastic egg cup. This is a good way to introduce her to another method of drinking.

Babies six months old and older may enjoy a dessert of fruit gel (fruit juice thickened with gelatine and cooled in the refrigerator—for a recipe, see page 186).

Freezing and thawing foods

Preparing food in large quantities and freezing it in small portions for your baby's future meals is a great time and money saver.

Containers for frozen food should be small; if they do not have lids, they should be placed in a large freezer bag before you put them in the freezer. An ice-cube tray that has been scalded with boiling water (or cleaned with a chemical sterilising solution as per instructions) is an ideal container; when frozen, pop the cubes of food into a freezer bag for long-term storage. Or you can simply spoon portions into small freezer bags.

It is important, when preparing the food for freezing, to take care with personal hygiene. Wash your hands before you begin, avoid touching pets when you are cooking, and do not re-use tasting spoons.

All frozen foods should:

- be maintained at a temperature of -18°C (0°F); you may need to check your freezer to ensure that it can maintain this temperature;
- be labelled with the date of storage;
- not be kept for longer than two or three months;
- be discarded once thawed; never refreeze food and then thaw it again.

Some foods, such as potato, do not freeze well on their own, and may need to be mixed in with other vegetables to be frozen successfully.

When thawing foods, keep the food covered. Thaw it in the fridge, or place it on a plate over a bowl of hot water or in a microwave on the 'defrost' setting. Heat the food just before serving it; food kept warm for prolonged periods is prone to bacterial contamination.

If the food is watery once thawed and mixed, it may be thickened with rice cereal, cottage cheese or potato.

Commercial baby foods

Most parents give their baby the occasional tin or jar of baby food. It can make life easier when travelling or visiting friends, or when life is too hectic to allow the preparation of fresh foods.

The advantages of commercial baby foods are that they are consistent in taste and texture; don't need to be stored in the refrigerator until opened; contain a wide selection of nutrients; and come in many varieties, including low sugar and salt varieties.

The disadvantages are that all the ingredients' flavours are blended together; most varieties are similar in taste and texture; they taste different from the fresh equivalent; they can be expensive; and their appearance is usually uninteresting.

THE INTRODUCTION OF SOLIDS

Packaged foods

The packaging and labelling of food can often be confusing. There are several important features you should check when purchasing packaged foods.

Check the 'use by' date—once this date has passed, the food may begin to deteriorate. Food with a shelf life of more than two years does not have to carry a date.

Storage instructions suggest the method of storage best suited to maintaining the quality of the product up to the 'use by' date.

Juices and baby foods in jars have a pop seal on the lid. If there is not a popping sound when you open the jar, you should return it to the point of purchase, as it is not fresh, or may have been opened already.

The 'net weight' is the actual weight of the product minus the packaging.

The ingredients must be listed in order of decreasing weight. Additives can be listed by category name and number (for example, 'stabilisers (407)') or by name (for example 'carrageenan'). Your early childhood health nurse or the National Health and Medical Research Council will be able to provide a list of additives and their corresponding numbers.

Safety

The kitchen can be a dangerous area for your baby when you are busy preparing a meal. Precautions to take include the following:

- Always put your baby down when you are cooking at the stove; spills and splashes can occur easily.

- A door barrier is a good idea to keep your baby out of the kitchen while you cook; she will still be able to see you but will be out of danger.

- Make a habit of turning saucepan handles inwards, for your own and your baby's safety, now and for later, when she is walking.

- Use curly cords on all electrical equipment, so that your baby cannot pull it down on top of herself.

- When feeding your baby, make sure she is safe. Never leave her unattended while she is eating finger foods. Make sure she is securely strapped into her feeding chair; the chair should be in good repair and stable.

- Remove tablecloths from tables, so that your baby cannot use them to drag food and equipment off the table or closer to herself.
- Her feeding equipment should be unbreakable and have no sharp edges.

Enjoyable mealtimes

It is important to make mealtimes a time of pleasure and not tension for either baby or parents. Especially after six months, babies like to help feed themselves, explore their food with their hands, and eat off other people's plates. To make life easier, accept that this behaviour is going to occur. Things that you can do to make mealtimes pleasurable for your baby include giving her a spoon so that she can help feed herself, offering finger foods and feeding her in an area where messes are easily cleaned up.

Vary the texture and appearance of the food, and offer realistic amounts of each type of food. Allow your baby to experiment with the feel of the food, maintain a sense of humour, and don't be offended if your baby does not appreciate your gourmet cooking. Whenever possible, adapt the family diet to suit your baby's needs, to save you extra cooking and possibly disappointment.

Feed your baby at regular intervals, so that she does not become cranky and tired by mealtime, and if possible feed her before the rest of the family eats so you can enjoy an uninterrupted meal. Give her finger food to enjoy while you are eating so that she will not feel left out.

Precautions to take when cooking and feeding

- Keep food preparation areas and equipment clean. Wash your hands before you start preparing food.
- Cooking equipment (except bottles and teats) does not need to be sterilised, but it should be washed in hot, soapy water and scalded with boiling water prior to use.
- Tasting spoons should not be re-used.
- Wash all fruit and vegetables thoroughly to remove dirt and pesticides. Try to avoid using pesticides in the kitchen, and if you do use them, cover foods while spraying.

THE INTRODUCTION OF SOLIDS

- Keeping food warm for prolonged periods can allow bacteria to multiply, causing food poisoning.
- Food left on your baby's plate after meals should be discarded, as it is very easy for contamination to occur from small amounts of your baby's saliva that have been transferred to the food.
- Fish should be double-checked for bones.
- When offering fresh vegetables or fruit to your baby, make sure they are not too crisp, with small pieces that could break off and cause her to choke. Lightly steaming vegetables will prevent this.
- Fruits with small seeds should not be offered to your baby—always take the seeds out first.
- If giving your baby bones to suck or chew, check for jagged edges and small, loose pieces of bone.
- Sweetened drinks should not be offered in a feeding bottle, as this is a major cause of tooth decay in small children.
- Check the temperature of all foods before offering them to your baby. Take special care with microwaved foods, as the outside may be cool but the centre may be extremely hot.

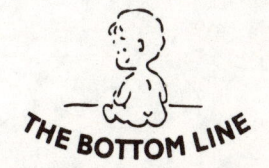

THE BOTTOM LINE

- Introduce one food at a time, and wait three days after introducing a new food to check for an allergic reaction.
- Never force your baby to eat.
- Where possible, feed her what the rest of the family is eating.
- Don't make elaborate meals for your baby when she is small.
- Feed the whole family a healthy diet.
- Don't add salt or sugar to baby foods—naturally occurring salts and sugars will be more than adequate.

CHAPTER 15

Recipes

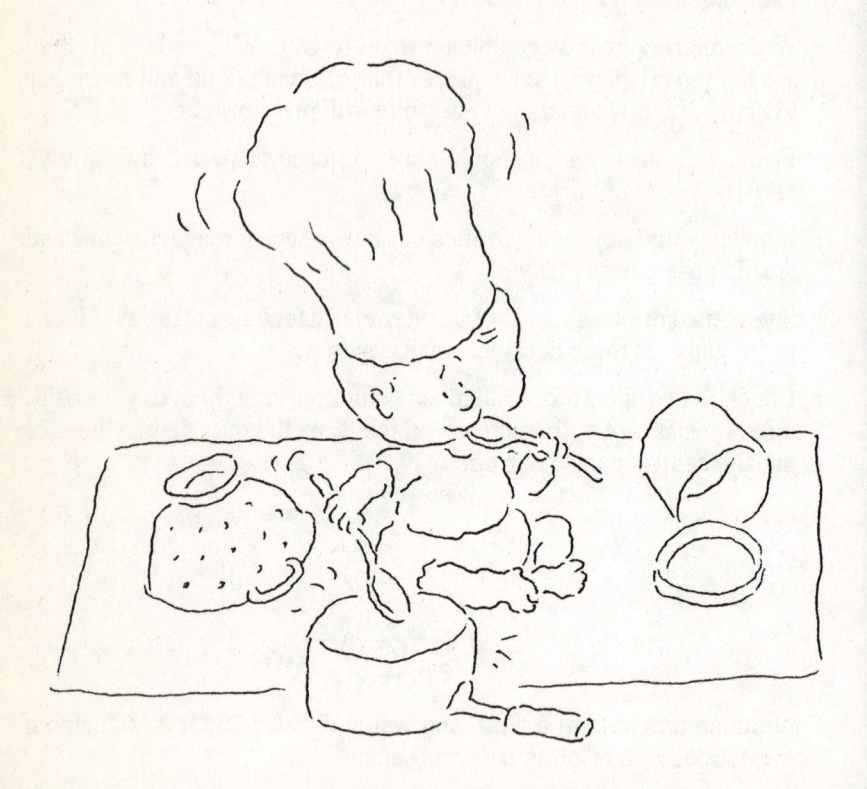

Before offering any of the meals suggested here, remember to check that your baby is not allergic to any of the ingredients.

RECIPES

Prune juice (3 months) — serve only to constipated babies (See Constipation, page 212).

For babies five to eight months old, put the prune pulp through a sieve. Older babies can be offered mashed prunes. The unused prune pulp can be stored in a sealed container in the refrigerator for forty-eight hours.

> *6 prunes, with the seeds removed*
> *250 mL (8 fl oz) water*

Bring the water to the boil. Add the prunes and simmer for ten minutes or until they are soft and can be easily mashed.

To microwave, place prunes and water in a microwave-proof dish and cook for 8 minutes on High.

Drain the juice from the pulp; it should be dark brown in colour. Strain the juice through a fine strainer and store it in a clean, covered bottle in the refrigerator.

Dilute it with cooled boiled water before offering it to your baby. See pages 178–9 for information on fruit juices.

Apple, apricot or pear purée (4 $^1/_2$ months)

Fruit contains natural sugar, so it does not require the addition of cane sugar. Remember that babies' taste preferences are different from adults', and they readily accept bland foods.

> *an apple, a pear or a few apricots (dried fruit may be used)*
> *enough water to just cover the fruit*

Peel, remove pit or core and slice fresh fruit. Dried fruit should be soaked in water overnight prior to cooking.

Place the fruit in a small saucepan with the water and bring it to the boil. Put a lid on the saucepan, turn the heat down and simmer for ten minutes or until the fruit is soft and easy to mash. Dried fruit may need to be cooked for a longer time.

To microwave, place fruit and water in a microwave-proof dish and cook on High for 5–6 minutes.

Drain and reserve the juice of the fruit, and mash the fruit with a fork. Add the reserved juice until the required consistency is achieved. Dilute leftover juice with equal amounts of cooled boiled water.

Creamed rice (5 months)

500 mL (16 fl oz) milk
  or 300 mL (10 1/2 fl oz) milk and 200 mL (7 fl oz) water
1/4 cup rice
a drop of vanilla essence

Wash rice well under cold running water, then drain it.

In a heavy-based saucepan, bring the milk, or milk-and-water mixture, to the boil. Add the rice and vanilla, and reduce heat to very low. Cover with a tight-fitting lid.

Cook the rice very gently, just barely simmering, to ensure that the rice does not stick to the bottom of the pan and burn, for about an hour, or until the mixture is a creamy consistency. Stir occasionally.

Fruit gel (5–6 months)

Do not offer this gel to your baby until he is accepting juice diluted to half-strength with water.

1 1/2 level teaspoons gelatine
125 mL (4 fl oz) boiled water
125 mL (4 fl oz) fruit juice

Dissolve the gelatine in the water. Add the fruit juice and mix well.

Pour the mixture into a bowl. Cover with a lid or plastic cling wrap.

Stand the bowl on a bench until cool, then store it in the refrigerator. The jelly is ready to eat when set.

Baked fish (6 months)

This is a good family meal; individual packages can be used for each piece of fish and seasoned to each family member's taste.

1 small piece of a fillet of a large fish such as gemfish (large fish usually have large bones that are easy to find and remove)
squeeze of lemon

Preheat the oven to 180°C (360°F)— moderate.

Wipe the fish with a clean cloth or a piece of kitchen paper to dry it, and place the fish on a piece of foil large enough to wrap it in. Squeeze a small amount of lemon juice over the fish, and wrap it in the foil.

Place the parcel on an oven tray and cook for 15–20 minutes.

When it is cooked, remove the fish from the foil. Take care not to burn yourself with the steam from inside the package. Remove any skin and bones from the fish. It is easy to check the fish for bones with your fingers. Flake the fish finely with a fork.

Serve the fish as it is, or combine it with vegetables, or mix it with a white sauce or well-cooked rice.

You can also microwave fish:

- Place fish piece on a microwave-proof dish.
- Cover loosely with plastic cling wrap, or put another plate on top, upside down.
- Cook on High for 4 minutes before testing to see if it is done; cook for longer if necessary. The length of time necessary will depend on the size of the fish piece.

Meat broth (6 months)

Meat broth can be offered to your baby as a clear soup or used as a base for leftover vegetables, pasta, rice or meats, depending on the age of your baby. Cook large enough quantities for a delicious winter meal for all the family.

The meat can be cut up finely or puréed with a food processor, blender or hand grinder.

Meat broth freezes well in an ice-cube container. Pop the frozen cubes out into a freezer bag and store them in the freezer compartment, labelled with the date.

1 lamb shank, or 100 g (3 oz) beef pieces or 1 chicken piece, such as a thigh, with the skin and fat removed
600 mL (21 fl oz) water

Place the meat and water in a saucepan and bring to the boil.

Reduce heat and gently simmer, covered, for about an hour and a half, or until the meat is separating from the bone. Alternatively, cook the meat in a pressure cooker for 30 minutes. You can also microwave the meat and water in a covered dish (plastic cling wrap will do as a cover, or use a dish with a lid). Cook on High for about 10 minutes. Check the liquid level at regular intervals and add extra fluid if necessary.

Strain the liquid into a bowl, allow it to cool, then refrigerate it until cold. Remove any fat that forms on top of the liquid.

Potato and cheese patties (6 months)

Other vegetables, salmon or tuna may be added to the mixture if desired.

1 potato
1 egg (yolk only, if your baby is under eight months)
2 tablespoons milk
1 tablespoon grated mild cheese
flour, breadcrumbs and olive oil

Boil or steam the potato. Beat the egg and milk together.

Combine the potato, egg and milk, and with a little flour form into patties and cover with breadcrumbs.

Fry in a little olive oil.

Yoghurt (6 months)

Plain yoghurt is a versatile food that can be used with savoury as well as sweet foods. Suggested additions are:

mashed vegetables
mashed, very ripe banana
prune pulp
grated raw apple
stewed apple or pear purée

Junket (6 months)

This is delicious served with fruit purèe.

$1/2$ junket tablet (vanilla flavour)
1 teaspoon cool boiled water
250 mL (8 fl oz) milk
$1/2$ teaspoon sugar

Crush the junket tablet in a medium-sized bowl and add the cool boiled water. Stir to dissolve the junket tablet.

Heat the milk and sugar in a small saucepan until warm. (This can be done in a bowl in a microwave oven.) Gradually pour the warm milk onto the dissolved junket tablet, stirring as you do so.

Pour the mixture into small moulds. (Don't use one large mould, as the mixture will separate once the surface has been cut.) Allow to set, then refrigerate.

Dried lentils or beans (7 months)

Cooked lentils or beans are an excellent addition to stews, casseroles, vegetables and soups. Precooked tinned beans are an alternative. If you are worried about any added salt in tinned beans, put them into a strainer and rinse them under running water before mashing.

It is important to boil legumes for a minimum of 15 minutes before adding them to casseroles or stews for further cooking, as they require prolonged cooking to make them suitable for your baby to eat. Before offering them to your baby, ensure that they can be easily mashed with a fork.

> $1/4$ cup lentils or beans
> 300 mL (10 fl oz) water
> additional 250 mL (8 fl oz) water

Soak the lentils or beans overnight in a covered bowl and the 300 mL water.

Drain the water off the lentils or beans, and combine the additional 250 mL water with the lentils or beans in a saucepan.

Bring to the boil and simmer for about 45 minutes, or until the lentils can be mashed easily with a fork, and all the water has been absorbed. Additional water may have to be added if further cooking is necessary.

Mash the lentils or beans with a fork.

Oatmeal porridge (8 months)

> 1 tablespoon rolled oats
> 60 mL (2 fl oz) water

Combine the rolled oats and water in a saucepan.

Bring to the boil, then turn the heat down and simmer gently for 5 minutes, stirring occasionally. Add extra water if necessary. Alternatively, microwave the mixture for 2–3 minutes on High, stirring occasionally.

Mix with formula or boiled cow's milk to serve.

Baked custard (8 months)

1 egg
2 teaspoons sugar
250 mL (8 fl oz) milk
vanilla essence

Preheat the oven to 150–180°C (300–350°F).

Beat the egg and sugar together. Add milk and vanilla essence, and mix well.

Pour into a greased baking dish.

Stand the dish in a larger tray containing hot water and bake slowly in the oven until set. Do not allow the custard to boil.

Home-made rusks (8 months)

These are a treat for babies who love to bite and chew.

Cut fingers of bread about 1 cm (½") in width. Place on an ungreased baking tray and crisp them in the oven on a very slow heat. Turn fingers once or twice to ensure that they become an even, golden colour. Cool them, then store in an air-tight tin. They will keep for five to seven days.

Always supervise your baby when he is eating rusks or any other finger foods.

Baby muesli (12 months)

1 tablespoon rolled oats
1 teaspoon ground almonds
1 teaspoon chopped sultanas
1 teaspoon finely chopped dried or fresh apricots
75 mL (2½ fl oz) water
Milk, formula or fruit juice

Combine all ingredients and cook in a saucepan on medium heat for 6 minutes, or until the mixture is soft. Alternatively, microwave the mixture for 5 minutes on High.

Add milk, formula or fruit juice and mix to a smooth consistency before serving.

Special Situations

CHAPTER 16

Travelling with your baby

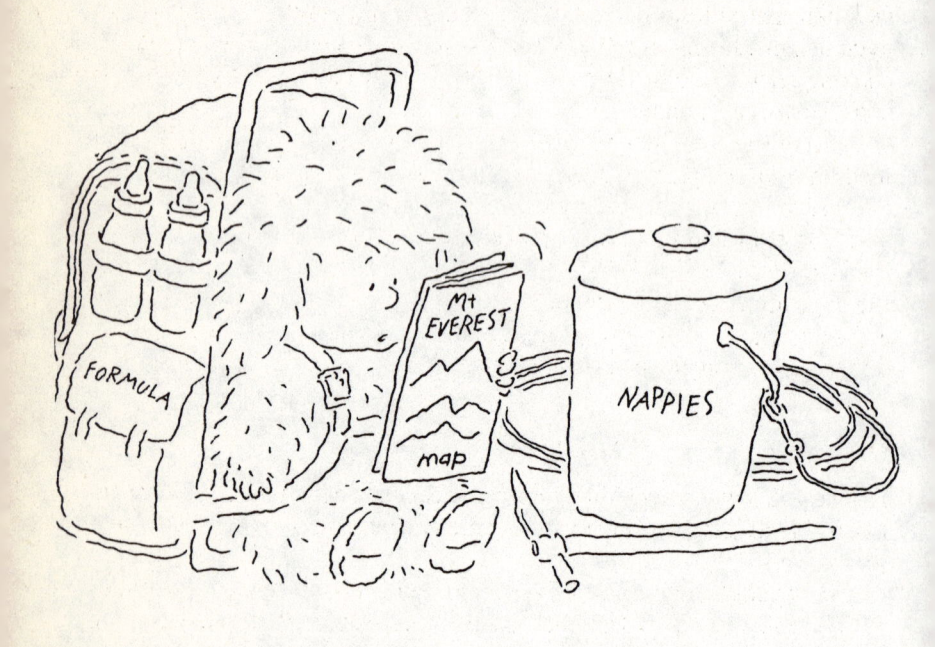

Now that you have a baby, you will find that going out resembles organising a trip to the Himalayas—unfortunately, without the Sherpas! Travelling with a baby requires more planning than travelling as a couple. The amount of planning required will be dependent on the length and destination of your trip, and the reason you are taking it.

Preparation is the key to success. Make lists of what you will take in the days leading up to your departure, and make all bookings and other arrangements well in advance, to avoid last-minute hitches. Try to strike a balance between catering for all eventualities and possible delays, and loading yourself down with unnecessary equipment, supplies and clothing.

Have realistic expectations of what you can do when you take a child along. The most restful holidays are usually those on which you travel to a single destination and stay there for the entire holiday. Your child can become used to her new bed, and there is time for a routine to become established. You may have to consider putting off some destinations or expeditions until your baby is older.

When working out suitable destinations, take into account the facilities that will be necessary for you to maintain basic standards of hygiene and cleanliness, that is: access to washing and drying facilities; cooking facilities, or at least the ability to heat bottles and baby foods; and a clean water supply.

During the time away from home, try to maintain your baby's usual feeding and sleeping patterns as much as possible, to minimise the disruptive effects of travel and to make her feel secure.

Most babies do not need to be sedated or have travel sickness medication to travel. In fact, in some babies this medication can have the opposite effect. If required, such medication should be prescribed by a doctor, and care should be taken that your baby does not become dehydrated because she is too sleepy to drink as much as usual.

Travelling by car

Before you leave, check that your car is packed well so that there are no loose objects that can become projectiles if you have an accident or have to stop suddenly.

Many parents travel at night so that their baby will sleep for a longer period. Take care that the parent who is driving does not become too tired, and stop every two hours to rest and refresh yourselves, for safety's sake. If you are travelling during the day, make frequent stops to change and feed your baby.

Protect your baby from the sunlight through the window. There are shade screens available for this purpose that allow the driver to see through the window; do not use a nappy or a towel.

Many small babies travel and sleep well in the car. If your baby is crying or becomes upset, stop the car and resettle her. A dummy is often helpful at these times, but glycerine, honey or any other sweetener should not be put on it to make the baby take it. It may help to have an adult sit in the back with your baby to stroke her and speak to her soothingly. Do not let your baby travel unrestrained in the car. *Carrying your baby in the front seat, especially on unfamiliar roads and in varying traffic conditions, is both unsafe and illegal.*

SPECIAL SITUATIONS

What to take

An approved **safety capsule or car seat** in which your baby can travel in safety is a legal requirement in all states of Australia. Ensure that it is fitted properly and that the straps hold your child firmly but not too tightly. See pages 237–8 for a list of things to check before buying a capsule or car seat.

Disposable **nappies** are a boon when you are travelling, as they are light and require no washing. If you are going to one destination where you will be staying for a week or so, and will have access to a washing machine, it is probably worthwhile taking **nappy buckets** and setting them up when you get there.

Try to take **clothing** that requires little ironing and dries quickly.

A **baby sleeping bag** (either an actual bag, or clothing with a bag built in) is a good investment unless you are going somewhere very hot. Even some places that are extremely hot during the day can be very cold at night, and babies do not maintain their body heat as well as adults do.

Depending on your baby's age, you will need to take a variety of quiet, soft **toys** to amuse her. Attach toys to the capsule with a short string so that you can retrieve them easily if your baby drops them.

If you are bottlefeeding, carry your **formula** in powder form and add it to cooled boiled water from a thermos flask or from a local café or milk bar. Make sure you shake the bottle well once you have added the powder, so that it is evenly distributed through the water. Do not carry your baby's milk formula already prepared while travelling, as it sours easily. You will also need to take **sterilising equipment**, if you are bottlefeeding. Sterilising tablets are handy.

A **large bag** to keep your baby's items together is a good idea, as is a **supply of plastic bags** to use for storage of soiled clothing, a clean wet washer and the collection of rubbish — be sure to keep plastic bags out of your baby's reach. A **clean wet washer** is useful for cleaning sticky hands and faces. It can also be used for your baby's forehead, to keep her cool on hot days and during long trips.

A **container of water** can be useful for cleaning up messes, and for you to drink from regularly if you are breastfeeding.

A supply of **toilet paper** is also handy for all the family, as many public toilets do not supply it; it is also useful when nappy-changing.

Caravan holidays

When you are on the road and towing your caravan, never leave your baby sleeping in the van. Besides being against the law, it is extremely dangerous, because of the risks of falling, fire, choking and lack of supervision.

Sometimes it may be difficult to keep your baby from crying. This is not easy to cope with in the confined space of a caravan, so do what you can to avoid it happening. Try to keep to your baby's usual routine as much as possible, and respond to any signs of tiredness.

Try to meet your neighbours at the caravan park and explain your situation. Ask them to come and see you if your baby's crying disturbs them. The responsibility then rests with them, and you need not worry about disturbing them unless they come to you. Let them know when your baby generally sleeps, so that they can perhaps keep their noise levels down at those times.

If you have a caravan in a permanent position in a caravan park, it might be wise to have the manager of the park move the van to an area away from other vans, if possible. You should not be too far from the laundry and bathroom facilities, however.

Be careful of the roadways in caravan and camping areas; often people are in the holiday spirit and are not as careful with road safety as they should be. Make sure you know where your baby is at all times. You may have to erect some kind of barrier at the caravan door to keep her safe.

Camping

When your baby is very small, camping may be a tiring form of holiday, as it may be difficult for you to maintain standards of hygiene in such matters as washing your hands, sterilising equipment and feeding your baby. You may wish to have a different type of holiday for a couple of years until your baby is bigger. However, small babies are easily transportable on short walks through the bush in carry pouches, and can find the experience stimulating. And, of course, any pastime that helps you to relax will be good for your baby, too. Preparation will make for a less stressful time, as will your care in protecting your baby from the sun and guarding against dehydration.

If you are bottlefeeding, you will have to take extra care with the preparation of your baby's formula. The formula should be made up only as needed, and used immediately.

Make sure that the drinking water is clean; you may need to use sterilising tablets to be sure. The taste of the water varies in different regions, so your baby may find the formula a little different and refuse it at first. Be patient; her hunger will usually overcome this reluctance.

You will need to take sterilising equipment with you for bottles and teats. Sterilising tablets are a good, compact method. You can also sterilise by boiling, but this is not as energy efficient.

Your baby will still need time on the ground to enhance her development. Make sure that you put her in a safe, open area and check for animals, snakes, spiders and other crawling insects. Put a blanket down for her to play on if the only open ground is hard dirt or scratchy grass.

It is always wise to know basic first aid and take a first aid kit with you when you are camping. Treatment for snake, spider and tick bites is given on page 256–7 and instructions on stocking a first aid kit are on page 226.

If you are bushwalking with your baby, be aware of the likelihood of ticks or leeches in the area, and check your baby and yourself at regular intervals during the walk and at the end of the day.

Ensure that your backpack fits correctly, and that the straps are adjusted so that you do not strain your back.

Make sure that your baby does not get sunburnt; put a hat and long-sleeved, cool clothing on her to prevent this happening. Put an SPF 15 plus sun-block on your baby's skin, and reapply it sparingly but frequently throughout the day. Take care that your baby does not become dehydrated if you are walking.

The sound of crying in the confined space of a tent can be trying for you to listen to. Try to keep to your baby's routine as much as possible so that she knows when it is an appropriate time to sleep, and do not ignore signs of tiredness. If she will not settle and the crying is disturbing you, pick her up and walk her up and down outside —her crying will not seem nearly as loud in the open air.

Train and coach travel

Deciding when to travel by train or coach can be difficult. Night travel is good if your baby is a good sleeper, but a wakeful child will be less of a problem during the day.

Try to travel on the lower deck of the coach if it is a double decker; there are fewer steps to negotiate if you need a drink, have to go to the toilet or need to disembark at every rest stop.

Wear shoes that are comfortable, so that you don't have to take them off. If the journey is long, your feet may swell and you may be unable to get your shoes back on at your destination.

If you are travelling alone, have your partner or a friend help you board the train or coach. He or she can hold your baby while you take your bags on board, find a seat and arrange your belongings, blankets and so on for the journey. This saves you having to juggle baby, bottles, clothes and other articles while the train or coach is moving. Try to be last on board to lessen the time spent in the confines of your seat. If possible, have someone meet you at your destination to help you disembark and carry your luggage.

Feeding your baby on the coach or train will sometimes help settle her; the combination of her usual breast or bottle and the movement and monotonous noise will often help put her to sleep.

Throughout your trip, carry your money on your person in a pocket that is not easily accessible from the aisle, particularly if you are travelling by train. You can then sleep in peace instead of having to keep a constant check on your baggage.

What to take

Only take what you cannot borrow at the other end. A **familiar soft toy** for your baby to take to bed may help settle her.

Take **one carry bag** that has lots of pockets and zippers. If possible, find a dark-coloured one so that dirt won't show. Carry bags make great footstools for long journeys and can be stored in the luggage rack above your head when you do not need them. Use the outside pockets for the articles you will need during the journey, and always use the same pockets for the same items, so that you can find them easily late at night, when the lights are out.

Take a **handful of plastic bags** with you. These are great for putting disposable nappies in, and for holding rubbish, soiled clothes and wet washers. A wet washer or hand towel is handy to help keep you and your baby clean and refreshed. Rinse it in fresh water when you have your rest stops, if you are going by coach.

Unless your baby is on a special **formula**, or you are going somewhere remote, you should be able to buy your formula on arrival. Only take a small amount of formula, in a small, sterilised plastic container, but take enough in case there is some kind of delay.

A **thermos flask of water** for making up formula, or for making coffee or tea for yourself, will keep hot on your journey. The staff on the train, or at the refreshment stops if you are travelling by coach, are usually quite happy to refill it for you. This saves you having to get out at road or rail-side stops to buy coffee or tea. A **container of cold water** is handy, especially if you are breastfeeding.

The same goes for **food**. Take some fruit or some prepared food for yourself to eat on the coach. Sometimes at rest stops, by the time you

SPECIAL SITUATIONS

have fed and changed your baby, you may not have much time to eat, and if you are on a train it can be difficult to get to the dining car or buffet with a small baby. It is important for you to eat.

A **sleeping bag** for your baby a is good idea, unless the weather is extremely hot, and it provides a familiar article for her at your destination. It won't fall off as easily as a blanket, and is warmer than the light blankets usually provided.

A **stroller** can be handy at bus and train stations; it can free your hands for luggage, as well as providing somewhere for your baby to sleep if you are delayed or waiting for transfers or connections.

Air travel

If your baby is very small, consider the benefits of flying, even though it is much more expensive. The main benefit is shorter travelling time. Of course, your finances may not stretch to air fares, or your destination may not be readily accessible by plane.

When booking your ticket, book directly with the airline you intend to travel on, if this is possible. This will avoid any misunderstanding about what facilities the airline provides for parents travelling with babies. Some airlines stipulate that each child under two years of age must be accompanied by an adult.

Many airlines cater for babies, allowing early seat allocation to ensure that parents are able to utilise bassinettes that are provided. These are suitable for babies up to about eight months of age. You will be allocated seats immediately behind the bassinette. Parents with babies may be allowed onto the plane earlier so that they have time to organise themselves and settle their babies before takeoff.

When you first board the plane, take the pillow and blanket from the overhead locker, so that you will not have to get them later.

Label your luggage clearly. Remove all old tickets at the end of each trip and have a large, bright, secure sticker or firmly tied piece of ribbon on the handle, so that you can find your luggage easily on the carousel at the other end of the trip, when you may be tired.

Many babies cry during takeoff and landing. Although this is distressing for you, it will help to equalise the pressure in your baby's ears. You can also give her a breastfeed, a bottle of cooled boiled water or a dummy to calm her at these times.

What to take

Some airlines provide food specially for babies. As a precaution, it may be wise to carry a small supply of baby food and formula, in case there is a mix-up and provision is not made for your baby, or if the cabin crew are busy — you can at least feed your baby until they are ready for you. The cabin crew will prepare your baby's formula and wash your bottles for you if you ask them.

Some airlines provide travel packs with disposable nappies, change lotion, cotton balls and tips, a washer, antiseptic towels and a bib. Larger planes have a special area with a baby change table.

Often airlines suggest that if you are breastfeeding you feed your baby in the washroom for privacy. As a breastfeeding mother, you have the right to feed where you are most comfortable, and where your baby is most settled. If you wish to feed in your seat and you are worried about privacy, you can cover your baby and breast with a poncho, shawl, large cardigan or airline blanket. This can also cut down on the visibility of any distractions for a baby older than six months, such as staff and passengers moving along the aisle.

Most babies do not need travel sickness medication or sedation to travel. Sedation presents a risk of dehydration, as your baby may not be awake to drink as much as usual. It also means that, if you are travelling through different time zones, when you arrive your baby may be wide awake at the times when you are most in need of sleep.

Your baby will need adequate fluids to help prevent dehydration and jet lag, just as you will. Drink a glass of fluid every hour, and avoid alcohol. Your baby will need her normal feeds and may have extra cooled boiled water or very diluted fruit juice.

Take something familiar for your baby to play with.

Dress your baby and yourself in loose, comfortable clothing. Take a jacket that you can take on and off easily for yourself, and a cardigan for the baby, as the air conditioning can be cold and draughty, especially on night flights. Ensure that the air flow valve is not directed on your baby.

It is wise to carry one change of clothes on the plane in case your baby needs a full change.

On some airlines you will have to stow your stroller with your luggage, so it is often helpful to have a carry pouch to put your baby in when you are getting on and off the plane and for transfers.

Water travel

Be extremely careful when taking your baby anywhere near water. *All* forms of water travel are potentially dangerous.

Sunburn is a hazard with water travel. Your baby will burn very easily, from the sunlight reflected off the water as well as from direct sunlight, and under the age of one year we recommend that you use a sun protection 15 plus. Dress your baby in light, long-sleeved clothing and a sunhat with a wide brim, and try to keep her in a sheltered area, and out of the sun altogether in the hottest period of the day.

Supervise your baby well, especially if she is mobile. Babies can move very quickly, and can get into difficulties or drown easily. A barrier around your boat is necessary if you frequently take your baby sailing. A safety harness and safety-standards approved life jacket are musts.

Help while holidaying

There are early childhood health centres in most towns around Australia. They have varying names; some are attached to the local hospital or community health centre, or are held in the local hall. Take your baby's record book with you when you travel; any of these centres will be pleased to see you and help you with any problems you may be having.

If you are travelling for any length of time, make sure that your baby's immunisations are kept up to date. Immunisation can be given by local general practitioners.

If you are travelling in an isolated area, be sure to let the local police station know where you are heading, and phone ahead to your next destination to let someone know when to expect you. Always check the condition of the road ahead, and drive with care.

If you are travelling in hot and humid conditions, be aware of the possibility of your baby getting a prickly heat rash. Some ways of avoiding and treating this condition are discussed on page 92.

Travelling overseas

Make sure that both your own and your baby's immunisations are up to date and take both of your immunisation records with you. Try to organise immunisations several weeks prior to travelling, so that you are not suffering from any reaction during the journey.

Take any medications needed for your baby or yourself with you. It is also wise to have a covering letter from your doctor, describing any illness or medical condition you are suffering from and the treatment you are undergoing.

Check, in advance if you can, the quality of the water supply at your destination. You may need to take sterilising tablets to make it drinkable for yourself and your baby.

Many baby formulas are available overseas. Often the one you use will be sold under a different name. Check with the manufacturing company before you go, so that you do not use up your baggage allowance with unnecessary extra formula. Initially, because the formula is made up with local water and may taste different, your baby may be reluctant to drink it. Be patient; she will soon get used to the taste. The same applies for new foods; watch for allergies.

If you are going away for several months or more, you may need to take fluoride tablets with you, as many countries do not have fluoride in their water supply.

Holidaying at home

Now that you have a baby, you may consider holidaying at home. Use the money you save to explore your own city, town or region.

Short day trips are less tiring. Go on picnics to national parks, the local river or the beach, but take care to protect yourselves against sunburn and practise water safety.

Spend time together as a family, going out walking or exploring your suburb or town. Ring your local tourist authority and find out about local sites you might visit, and go to museums and galleries.

Do minimal housework at holiday time. Concentrate on relaxing and enjoying yourself and getting to know your family better. Buy takeaway foods occasionally, or foods that you do not usually eat or prepare, for their novelty value and to save you cooking.

Arrange babysitting for an evening, and go out to dinner or the movies.

Extra equipment

A worthwhile investment if you are planning a lengthy trip is a **portable cot**. Most babies enjoy a change in their sleeping environment, but feel secure if their cot is familiar. These cots are also useful when you are visiting, or are leaving your baby at someone's home.

As with all baby equipment, the price of portable cots seems to be variable, depending on the features, style or colour of the cot. Regardless of the cost, look for the following safety features.

The cot should be stable and not collapse if your baby stands up in it. Any hinges should not be in a position where they can scratch or pinch your baby's fingers. If the cot is a painted one, the paint should be non-toxic. If it is wooden, the rails should be smooth. The base should be

SPECIAL SITUATIONS

secure, and there should not be a gap between the mattress and the base that could trap your baby's head or limbs. You should buy the mattress that is made to fit the cot.

You may also want to buy a **portable baby chair**. There are several types on the market. Check that the one you are considering purchasing will fit onto most tables or benches. Do not attach it to a single pedestal table, as the weight of your baby may overbalance the table. Do not leave your baby unsupervised in the chair.

Many restaurants now provide highchairs or booster seats. It is worthwhile checking to see if this service is available before taking your child out to dinner. At the same time, ask if the restaurant can seat your family in a secluded area, especially if you are self-conscious about breastfeeding in public, or are worried about your children disturbing other diners.

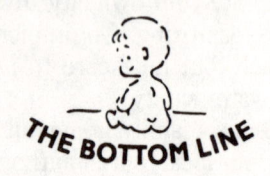

THE BOTTOM LINE

- Preparation is the key to success.
- For a holiday that both you and your baby enjoy, you need to prepare thoroughly and well in advance.
- Know your limits and do not have unrealistic expectations; holidays can be hard work.
- Have a first aid kit handy, and be aware of the possible dangers to your child, including sunburn.
- Do not automatically assume that your baby will suffer from motion sickness or require sedation.
- Maintain your standards of hygiene, and keep your baby's feeding equipment sterilised.
- Maintain your baby's sleeping and feeding routines.

CHAPTER 17

Caring for your sick baby

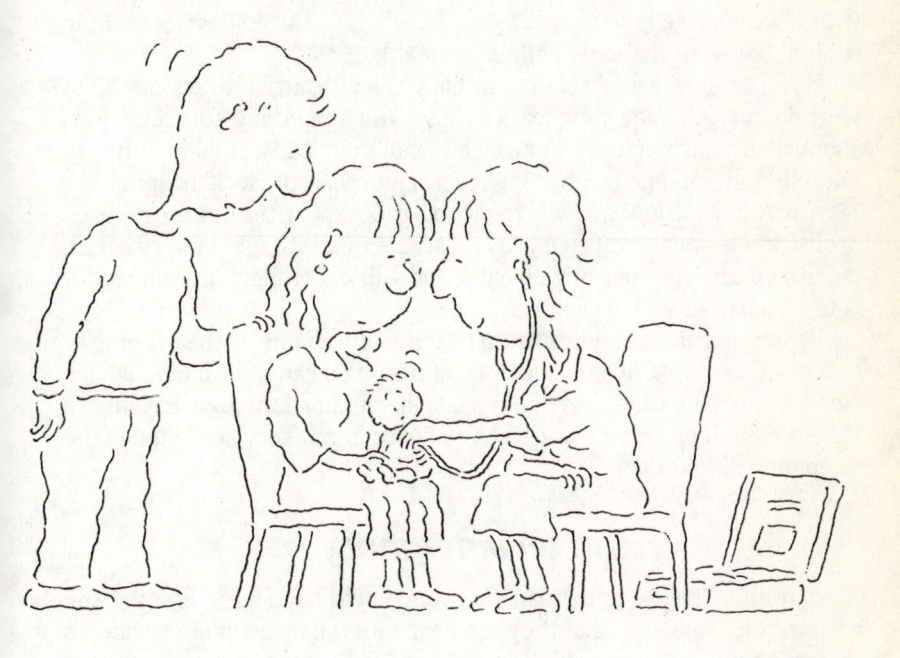

An unwell baby places a great deal of stress on his parents. In most cases babies become ill quickly and recover just as rapidly, but it may take parents days to recover from the anxiety caused by the illness, and the tiredness resulting from sleepless nights.

Parents should take extra care of themselves and one another during such stressful times, taking turns at sleeping if the baby needs constant care. Make sure that you both continue to eat adequately and well. Prioritise the housework, and don't worry about doing tasks that will wait. The most important thing to do is to stay in touch with each other and to share your feelings about what is happening and how you are coping.

SPECIAL SITUATIONS

How to get help

It is important for every family to have a local doctor in whom they feel confident. You should feel free to ask questions about your children's health and behaviour, no matter how simple or how silly you think the questions sound. The on-going care of a family by one doctor helps build rapport and makes diagnosis of illness simpler. Another major aspect of your doctor's role is to monitor your baby's growth and development in conjunction with the early childhood health nurse.

If you are concerned about your baby's health, a visit or phone call to your doctor will allay your fears or give you something concrete to do about it. If your doctor is unavailable, call your early childhood health nurse for advice, and referral if necessary, or visit the local hospital.

Always act if you are worried. You can expect that in most cases health professionals will give you reassurance and straightforward advice on how to care for your unwell baby, and will understand how difficult it is to be a parent with a sick baby.

Babies and small children often become unwell during the evening or at night. Paediatric hospitals and local hospitals can offer phone advice services for such cases. Advice can also be obtained through Tresillian's Parent Help Line service or residential parentcraft services listed in the telephone directory.

In an emergency

All parents of babies and small children should have basic first aid and resuscitation skills, so that they can deal with the many minor accidents that will happen to their children and cope with any major accident that occurs. See pages 255–6 for emergency resuscitation instructions.

Classes in first aid and resuscitation are run by organisations such as the Red Cross Society and the St John Ambulance Association. Information can be obtained about the courses through their headquarters in each capital city. See page 248 for telephone numbers.

Make a list of all the emergency numbers you may need on the chart on page 14 of this book. Photocopy it and put it in a prominent place by the telephone.

Medication

Take great care when giving your child medicines or applying creams and ointments. Only give medications that have been **specifically**

prescribed for your baby. Do not use other people's medications.

Give the **dosage as recommended** by your doctor, or, in non-prescription medicines, as advised on the container. The dosage is usually dependent on the child's age—check this with your chemist. If you are in doubt about the dosage, contact your doctor.

Complete the course of medicine as advised by the doctor even if your baby's condition appears to be improving. If your baby's condition is not improving with medication, ring or return to your doctor for advice.

Careful storage of medicines is important to prevent them deteriorating. Store them out of direct sunlight, or in a refrigerator if this is recommended. After opening bottles and tubes, ensure that the lid or cap is firmly replaced. Always store medicines out of the reach of children and if possible in a cupboard with a childproof lock.

Check the **'use by' date** on medicines, and discard them if they are out of date. Discard leftover medication when the illness is over unless it is a multi-purpose medication such as paracetamol.

When applying **creams or ointments**, make sure your baby does not get cream on his finers, as he may suck them later and suffer an allergic reaction. Do not give the cream container to the baby while you are applying the cream, as he will probably put it straight into his mouth. All creams, lotions, ointments and medicines are potentially harmful.

If medication for pain or fever is needed, always give **paracetamol** unless otherwise specified by your doctor, as children have difficulty tolerating aspirin. Unless advised otherwise by your doctor, only give babies medicines **specifically developed for paediatric use.**

How to give medicines

Babies are usually given medicines in the form of liquid or syrup. To make sure you are giving the right dosage of the medicine:

- Read the label and the instructions on the bottle.

- Check that you are giving the right medicine in the specified amount, at the correct time.

- Shake the bottle well.

- Pour the correct amount into a medication measuring cup or plastic medicine dropper. These are available at most chemists.

- If your baby vomits, or develops a rash or a wheeze soon after taking the medicine, check with the doctor before giving him another dose.

SPECIAL SITUATIONS

The method you use to offer your baby the medicine will be dependent on his age and mobility, and your skilfulness. If your partner is available to help you, one of you can hold your baby while the other administers the medicine. If you are on your own and are having difficulty administering the medication, we suggest that you wrap your baby firmly in a cot sheet and prop him on your lap at a 45-degree angle. Use a plastic medicine dropper to administer the liquid. Most babies will suck the medicine out of the dropper, or it can be gently squeezed so that the medicine runs down the inside of your baby's cheek. Avoid squeezing the dropper too vigorously or directing it down your baby's throat, as this may make him gag.

A medicine cup can be used for an older baby, but take care that your baby does not dribble too much of the medicine out of the corners of his mouth. Never put your baby's medicine into his feed: he may start to refuse bottles, or he may not finish the feed, so that the full dosage of medicine is not given.

How to apply creams, ointments and lotions

The application of creams, ointments or lotions can be a messy business. The following suggestions may help.

Always **wash your hands** before touching any reddened or broken skin, or any equipment that will come into contact with this area of skin. This will limit the chances of the area becoming infected.

Remove old traces of creams or ointments with a small amount of organic oil, such as olive or almond, prior to the next application.

Always **read the directions for use** on the container and follow them carefully; if prescribed by your doctor use only as directed.

Thick ointments, such as zinc and castor oil, work by sitting on the skin surface and providing a protective barrier. They can stain your baby's clothing and nappies; use a clean piece of old sheeting or soft cotton fabric, cut to the size of the area to be covered (if this is a large area, two or three smaller pieces are advised for ease of placement).

The ointment can be applied directly to this piece of cloth with a clean butter knife or spatula, or a cloth-wrapped finger. Gently dab the affected skin surface with the ointment, then lay the piece of material over the affected area. This will lower the risk of infection to your baby, and cause him less pain than trying to rub the ointment on with your fingers. The material will help keep the cream in place and protect your baby's clothing.

This method works well in the nappy area, or where clothing fits snuggly. In areas such as behind the ear or in the chin creases, apply the ointment with the piece of material, but do not cover the area with the cloth.

Creams are much lighter in consistency and are usually meant to be rubbed into the skin. Always apply them sparingly, as you can add more if necessary.

Lotions are usually liquid in consistency. Some are simply dabbed on and left; others should be rubbed into the skin. Cottonwool or old cotton material can be used to dab lotion onto the skin.

Creams, ointments and lotions can be expensive to buy. If a special type or brand of cream is suggested to you by your doctor or early childhood health nurse, ask if one of the creams that you already have in your medicine cupboard will give you the same results. Before applying it, check that it is not past its expiry date.

Feeding your unwell baby

Babies usually adjust their appetites according to how they are feeling. Don't force an unwell baby to eat solid foods; offer him only small amounts of food, unless otherwise advised by your doctor. Allow him to eat what he wants (avoiding fried or very rich foods, of course).

It is more important that he maintain adequate fluid levels. Continue to breastfeed or offer the usual milk formula, unless advised otherwise by your doctor. Breastmilk is easy to digest and has protective qualities, and only on *very* rare occasions does breastfeeding need to be ceased altogether. Additional fluid may be advised in the form of cool boiled water.

High temperature

A high temperature is usually the first sign that your baby is unwell. The normal body temperature is around 37° Celsius (99.5°F). It is advisable to maintain a baby's temperature between 36.4°C and 37.2°C (97.5–99°F). Contact your doctor for advice if your baby's temperature is higher than 37.5°C; it is dangerous for a baby to have such a high temperature, as it puts him at risk of having fits (convulsing).

Babies react differently to a high temperature—some become unsettled, flushed and fretful, while others become pale and lethargic. A thermometer is an inexpensive piece of equipment that is essential for all households, as you will be asked what your baby's temperature is if you ring a health professional for advice.

SPECIAL SITUATIONS

To take your baby's temperature:

- Shake the thermometer until the mercury is contained in the bulb.

- Never place a mercury thermometer in your baby's mouth (he may break it by biting on it) or in his anus, as you may injure him. Place the bulb of the thermometer under your baby's armpit, making sure that it is held between two folds of his skin and not just his clothing.

- Hold the thermometer in place by applying gentle pressure to your baby's upper arm; this can be done while cuddling your baby on your lap. Keep it in place for a full minute.

- If the temperature reading does not correspond with your feelings about your baby's temperature, replace the thermometer and leave it for a further minute.

- After use, rinse the thermometer in cold, soapy water, and return it to its container for safe-keeping.

There are other types of thermometers available, including pressure strips that are held against the baby's forehead—these are not very accurate—and digital thermometers, which are expensive, but may be a worthwhile investment. To reduce a raised temperature, a combination of techniques can be used:

- Give your baby a bath in lukewarm water (neither cool nor too warm). Do not use cold water, as this will cause the blood vessels to contract, when you want them to dilate, to promote cooling.

- Dress your baby in natural fibres, such as cotton, which absorbs perspiration and is more comfortable for an unwell baby than synthetic fabrics.

- Do not strip your baby completely; always leave him dressed in a nappy and a cotton singlet, to absorb any perspiration. A loosely tucked cotton sheet over your baby in his cot or bassinette is usually more comfortable for him than no covering at all.

- Place your baby in a cool room, but out of draughts or breezes from fans. Babies can chill very easily.

- A dose of infant paracetamol can be effective in lowering your baby's temperature and can provide relief from associated pain or discomfort. Give no more than three doses in twenty-four hours and at a maximum every four hours, unless ordered otherwise by your doctor.

If your baby's temperature does not return to and stay below 37.5 degrees Celcius, we would advise you to seek your doctor's advice. A high temperature is only a symptom of illness, not an illness in itself. The underlying cause may need treatment before your baby's condition improves.

Vomiting

Many babies vomit at feed time. The amount varies from only a dribble (often called a posset) to a large proportion of the feed. If your baby vomits regularly at feed time, but is gaining weight and is alert, there is usually no cause for concern; some babies have a weak valve between the oesophagus and the stomach. This type of vomiting (sometimes called 'oesophagal reflux') is usually self-limiting and will diminish as your baby starts to sit up, causing the valve to strengthen. If any treatment is necessary, it should only be recommended by your doctor, as other causes of vomiting will have to be excluded.

Methods we use at Tresillian to limit or alleviate feed-time vomiting include the following:

- Play with your baby prior to a feed, and handle him gently after a feed.

- Prop your baby's bassinette or cot up by placing a rolled-up towel or pillow under the mattress at the head of the bassinette. Do not raise the mattress too high or your baby will fall out. For a cot, place bricks or large blocks under the two legs at the head end, making sure that the cot is stable and will not roll off the blocks.

- Slow down your baby's feeding. Use a slower teat if bottlefeeding. If breastfeeding, express for a few minutes prior to the commencement of the feed, which will help take the initial gush of milk away. See pages 138–9 for guidelines on expression.

- Check the formula preparation method and the strength of formula if you are bottlefeeding your baby. If formula is made up incorrectly it can cause vomiting.

- Offer small and frequent drinks of breastmilk or formula, rather than large feeds at long intervals.

Your baby should be examined by your doctor if the vomiting is causing you concern, even if your baby appears to be thriving. Consult your doctor about vomiting if your baby:

SPECIAL SITUATIONS

- does not normally vomit
- has a high temperature
- has diarrhoea
- is abnormally sleepy or lethargic
- seems to be suffering pain or discomfort
- is unsettled or difficult to settle
- is refusing the breast, bottle and/or solid foods
- is not having as many wet nappies during the day
- is producing vomit with an offensive smell, or that contains bile (yellow–green) or blood, or
- is forcefully vomiting.

Do not give your baby any medication for the vomiting until you have obtained advice from your doctor.

If vomiting is excessive or prolonged, your baby's skin, especially in his chin and neck folds, may need special care. At regular intervals, wash it with warm water, and a little soap if his skin is not dry, then rinse. Apply a light protective covering of cream such as zinc and castor oil, sorbolene and glycerine or petroleum jelly.

Place a thick towel under your baby's pillow case to protect the mattress. *Never* use a piece of plastic, as it introduces a real risk of suffocation.

Diarrhoea

There are a great many variations in the bowel motions of babies (see page 93 for general remarks). Diarrhoea is usually described as loose, frequent bowel motions. They can have an offensive smell. The bowel motion can be watery, mucous and/or contain particles of blood.

If there is any variation from your baby's normal bowel motion, you should seek advice from your doctor or early childhood health nurse. *Diarrhoea can be a life-threatening condition in babies and small children, so always see a doctor,* as treatment of the cause and symptoms should be commenced as soon as possible.

There are many reasons why diarrhoea may occur, including an infection, such as gastroenteritis; an intolerance or allergy to a food or a type of milk; or a medication, such as an antibiotic.

CARING FOR YOUR SICK BABY

It is important that you do not give your baby any medication to stop the diarrhoea, as you will then no longer have a reliable indicator of the improvement or deterioration of his condition.

Gastroenteritis (infection of the gut) has been one of the major causes of death in babies in past decades. Simple precautions can protect your baby from this illness:

- Good personal hygiene. Wash your hands after using the toilet and before handling food or bottles.

- Continued breastfeeding if possible, for the antibodies that breastmilk provides.

- Sterilisation of all baby's feeding equipment and dummies (see pages 164–5 for directions).

- Adequate, cold storage of your baby's food and bottles (see pages 139, 161–2 for guidelines).

If your baby does develop diarrhoea, contact your doctor for advice. Avoid contact with other babies and small children, until you know that your baby's condition is not infectious. Take care with the disposal or washing of soiled nappies. Remove any faeces from disposable nappies before putting them out with the garbage. (Be sure to check that disposal of these nappies in the household garbage is legal in your state). Rinse soiled nappies thoroughly before soaking or washing, and wash them separately from other clothing. Continue good hand-washing and hygiene practices.

You will probably need to protect your baby's buttocks, as frequent bowel motions can easily result in rashes. Frequent nappy changes will be required.

Avoid the use of commercial nappy-change lotions at this time, as these can irritate any raw skin. Instead, wash your baby's buttocks with warm water and unperfumed soap. If the skin is damaged (red, raw or bleeding), the use of olive oil or sorbolene and glycerine to remove any adhered bowel motion may be less painful for your baby than simple wiping, and will not irritate the skin.

At every change, protect the skin after washing it by applying a protective cream, such as zinc and castor oil or petroleum jelly. Use zinc and starch powder if the skin's surface is broken. Cover the area with cotton cloth to protect your baby's clothing and keep the cream against his skin.

SPECIAL SITUATIONS

Dehydration

There are many possible causes for a baby becoming dehydrated. These may include gastroenteritis, or any illness with associated vomiting and/or diarrhoea, and heat exhaustion. Heat exhaustion can occur if you leave your baby in a hot car or the hot sun for even a short time. Signs of dehydration are lethargy, drowsiness, a dry mouth, sunken eyes, a sunken soft spot (fontanelle), and a period of twelve to twenty-four hours without passing urine.

It is important to seek a doctor's assistance urgently if your baby becomes dehydrated, as his life is at risk.

Constipation

Constipation is a condition relating to the consistency (hardness) of bowel motions, not their frequency. It is extremely rare for a fully breastfed baby to be constipated, but constipation may occur once solid food has been introduced into his diet. Causes of constipation may include incorrect formula preparation (formula made too strong), an inadequate fluid intake, an unbalanced diet, or illness.

If you are bofflefeeding your baby and he is constipated (that is, passing hard, dry bowel motions), check that you are making up his formula with the correct proportion of water to formula. Additional fluid in the form of cool boiled water or diluted fruit juice can be given to a constipated baby; remember to check for allergies if your baby has not previously been given fruit juice. The juice drained off stewed prunes can be effective (see page 185 for recipe), but you should take care, as juices can cause your baby to have loose bowel motions.

If your baby is on solid foods, check the type and amount of the foods you are offering him. If he is taking a variety of foods, increase the proportion of fruit and vegetables in his diet—remember to check for allergies before offering new types. Prune pulp can be effective in softening your baby's bowel motions. Start by offering him a teaspoonful, once a day, then gradually increase to two tablespoons (eight teaspoons) over a period four days.

Try using relaxation techniques, baby massage, bathing and gentle exercises to relax your baby. See pages 69–75 for guidelines.

Only rarely are laxatives or suppositories necessary; they should only be used after consultation with your doctor. Do not put pieces of soap or any other objects in your baby's anal passage. This does not treat the cause of the constipation, and may tear or damage your baby's anus.

CARING FOR YOUR SICK BABY

Nappy rash

It is common for babies, even those with the most caring of parents, to develop angry, reddened areas of skin under their nappies. There are many causes of nappy rash, including the following:

- The skin being in constant contact with urine.

- Sensitive skin — some babies are more prone to developing nappy rash than others.

- The excessive use of soaps, especially perfumed soaps; these can wash away the natural oils that protect the skin.

- Detergents, softening agents or sterilising agents used when you wash your baby's nappies may be too harsh for his skin. Rinse nappies thoroughly after washing. See page 94 for nappy-washing instructions.

- The warm moist conditions created by the use of plastic pants or disposable nappies are ideal for the development of skin infections. An infection will aggravate any reddened area inside the nappy.

Occasionally none of these causes will apply, but your baby will still be suffering from a rash. If your baby's nappy rash is difficult to treat with simple skin care, by changing your nappy washing method or by discontinuing the use of plastic pants, pilchers or disposable nappies, seek the advice of your early childhood health nurse or doctor. Many persistent nappy rashes are due to a thrush (fungal) infection, which will need special treatment.

Prevention is far better than cure, so try to avoid or limit the effects of nappy rash by changing your baby at regular intervals and washing his buttocks at least once a day, and after each bowel motion. Depending on the condition of his skin, this can be done with soap and water or olive oil.

Apply a water-resistant cream, such as zinc and castor oil or petroleum jelly, to your baby's buttocks, especially if he is sleeping through the night. Avoid using plastic pants, plastic-lined pilchers or disposable nappies for long periods; perhaps use them only when you are going out. When at home, use double cloth nappies to lessen the amount of moisture soaking through onto your baby's clothes.

Take care that nappies are washed and rinsed thoroughly. If you are using a chemical nappy sterilising solution, check that you are using it as directed, and make sure you rinse the nappies well.

Thrush

Thrush (monilia) is caused by a fungal infection (*Candida albicans*). It can occur virtually in any area that is constantly moist and warm. The main areas in which it affects babies are in the mouth and on the buttocks.

Thrush is a normal inhabitant of the bowel and it is not harmful if it stays in the bowel. If our body's chemical balance is changed or there is a breakdown of skin tissue and contamination from another source, thrush can rapidly multiply in areas in which it normally would not survive. Potential causes of thrush developing and being transferred are:

- Changes in the hormonal balance in the body.
- Changes in the body's chemical balance due to the taking of antibiotics.
- Inadequate sterilisation of bottles, teats and feeding equipment.
- Putting thrush-contaminated fingers into your own or your baby's mouth.
- Breastfeeding—your baby can pick up thrush if you have a thrush infection on your nipples.
- Using plastic pants or disposable nappies for prolonged periods if your baby has nappy rash. The plastic causes the nappy area to be constantly warm and moist, ideal conditions for thrush to multiply.
- If you either had vaginal thrush when your baby was born, or have a thrush infection currently, contamination may occur.

The appearance of a thrush infection in your baby will vary depending on the site. In the mouth, it looks like white milk curds, but they are difficult to remove, and if you do remove them they leave a red raw area. In the nappy area thrush usually looks like a fine, pimply rash, starting around the anus. If your baby has a nappy rash that will not improve, it may be infected with thrush. Always get a doctor or early childhood health nurse to check the rash. On other areas of the body, suspect a thrush infection if skin cracks or wounds will not heal and remain moist and inflamed. Vaginal thrush will cause a thick white discharge from your vagina, and you will probably have feelings of discomfort and vulval irritation.

Thrush is easily transferred from one area to another, so washing your hands before touching your baby or any equipment that will go into your baby's mouth is your best defence.

Seek the advice of your doctor or early childhood health nurse if you suspect that you or your baby has any thrush infection. It is important to treat the source of the thrush as well as the symptoms, to ensure that it does not return.

Cradle cap

Cradle cap (seborrhoeic dermatitis), the development of greasy, yellowish scales on your baby's scalp, is a common problem. There are many reasons why cradle cap can occur, but the two most common reasons are not rinsing the soap or shampoo out of your baby's hair adequately, and not massaging or stimulating your baby's scalp adequately. In some cases, cradle cap persists, no matter how careful you are with your baby's hair care, and the cause is never found.

To treat cradle cap, gently massage sorbolene and glycerine cream, or olive oil, into your baby's scalp and leave it overnight, or for one hour prior to washing your baby's hair. This will soften it, and assist in the removal of the scales—this can be done by gently combing with a fine-toothed comb or face washer.

Wash your baby's hair regularly. If you are using sorbolene and glycerine, water is all that is necessary. If you are using oil, you may need to use a small quantity of a mild shampoo or non-perfumed soap. Rinse well.

Massage your baby's scalp well with the flats of your fingers when washing his hair, especially the area over his fontanelle, as this is where cradle cap occurs in most babies.

Use a soft brush to brush your baby's hair when it is dry; this will help to stimulate his scalp. Do not pick at or rub the scalp too vigorously to remove the scales, as this will cause bleeding and a potential site for infection.

There are several products available to treat cradle cap, usually in the form of a lotion or shampoo. These treatments have been found to be effective by some parents.

The eyebrows and the skin folds of your baby's ears may also be affected by cradle cap. The treatment of these areas is the same as for his scalp—moistening the scales, then gently massaging the area.

The common cold

The common cold affects most families at least once every year. Babies tend to be more susceptible to viruses, as they have an immature immune system. There is not much you can do to protect your baby from

SPECIAL SITUATIONS

contracting a cold, as the viruses are usually airborne; most babies have three colds within their first year of life.

Babies tend to have very generalised symptoms when they have a cold: a high temperature (above 37.5°C—99°F), a runny and/or stuffy nose, sneezing, watery eyes, lethargy (a sleepy, dull appearance), a lack of appetite, perhaps some difficulty feeding due to a blocked nose, and irritable behaviour.

Colds usually don't require any special treatment, but see your doctor if you are concerned about your baby's health. Relief of the associated symptoms will make your baby feel more comfortable.

It is important to lower your baby's temperature. (See pages 207–9 for suggestions.)

If your baby's eyes are watery, gently wipe them with cooled boiled water, wiping from the inside of the eye outwards. This takes any debris away from the tear duct.

If your baby's appetite is poor, offer him small, frequent feeds. Allow him to take as much or as little as he wishes. Keep a watchful eye on the number of wet nappies he produces. See page 212 if you are worried about dehydration.

Dress your baby in comfortable, loose clothing and avoid overdressing. Gentle handling and extra cuddles will help soothe your irritable baby. Remember, the grizzling or irritable behaviour is your baby's only way of telling you how uncomfortable he is feeling.

A stuffy nose can make feeding difficult, and your baby may pull off the breast or bottle frequently to breathe through his mouth. It is best to seek your doctor's advice before using nose drops, as they may cause damage to the lining of your baby's nasal passages. Any mucus crusts that form around the nose can be gently removed with warm water and a twisted piece of cotton wool—don't use cotton tips for this task, as he may move, and you could damage his nose.

You may notice mucus in your baby's bowel motions (or in his vomit, if he possets). This is usually mucus that has been swallowed. Babies are unable to blow their noses or cough any excess mucus up. If there is blood mixed with the mucus, see your doctor.

The common cold usually lasts from two to ten days. It is important to see your doctor for advice if your baby develops a persistent cough, if his temperature remains high or if there is any significant vomiting or diarrhoea.

CARING FOR YOUR SICK BABY

Middle ear infection

Babies and small children are prone to middle ear infections (otitis media) as they have short, straight Eustachian tubes (tubes that run from the middle ear to the throat). These tubes lengthen and change shape as the child grows, so that the risk of middle ear infections lessens.

A middle ear infection is a painful condition. Your baby may be unsettled and wake more frequently at night as a result of it. Older babies may pull at their ears. There may be an associated high temperature and/or a respiratory tract infection.

If your baby is displaying uncharacteristic irritable behaviour and waking more frequently at night, if he develops a high temperature or has a persistent respiratory tract infection, you need to seek advice from your doctor.

Cot death

Cot death (Sudden Infant Death Syndrome) is one of the most tragic and feared events for many parents. There are many theories about what causes otherwise thriving babies to die suddenly, none of which has been proven as the main or only reason. However, we do know that putting your baby to sleep on his side or back, breastfeeding, avoiding overwrapping and not smoking near your baby significantly lessens the risk of SIDS.

If a cot death occurs, parents need to be aware of the support and assistance that is available. The Sudden Infant Death Association is an organisation set up specifically to provide support and advice to parents by other parents who have lost a child to cot death. See pages 249–50 for phone numbers. All doctors and early childhood health nurses have an understanding of the issues that parents will be concerned about and need to address.

It is important that parents do not feel guilty or blame themselves for their baby dying from a cot death. This type of infant death has occurred since biblical times. Parents should be given an opportunity to say goodbye to their baby; this will be distressing at the time, but will help them adjust to the reality of their baby's death. The baby's mother and father should support and communicate with each other during this distressing period to ensure that neither is blaming her or himself for the death of the baby.

Individuals grieve in different ways, and the grieving process cannot be rushed. Parents need to be aware that the other children in the family will be deeply affected, even if they appear not to be concerned or upset about the baby's death. Parents should make sure that the other children do not blame themselves for the death of the baby; they may sometimes have wished the baby dead and believe that their wish was responsible for his death. There are many ways that small children react after a death in the family; these can include a need to imitate in their play what occurred at the time of the baby's death, telling stories about what happened, and exhibiting attention-seeking or clinging behaviour.

If you find yourself overly concerned about the possibility of cot death, discuss your fear with your early childhood health nurse or doctor.

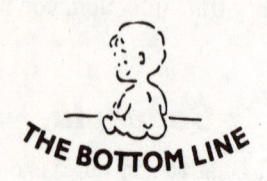

THE BOTTOM LINE

- Take your baby to the doctor immediately if he has diarrhoea, if he vomits in a way that is abnormal for him, if he appears to be dehydrated or if he has a raised temperature that will not drop below 37.5°C (99.5°F) after simple treatment.
- Breastfeed your baby if possible.
- Put your baby to sleep on his side or back.
- Avoid overwrapping.
- Avoid smoking near your baby.
- Keep a list of emergency numbers by the telephone.
- Learn first aid and resuscitation skills.
- Take care of one another, so you don't become unwell yourselves.
- Seek your doctor's or early childhood health nurse's advice, even with concerns that you may feel are trivial.

CHAPTER 18

Leaving your baby in care

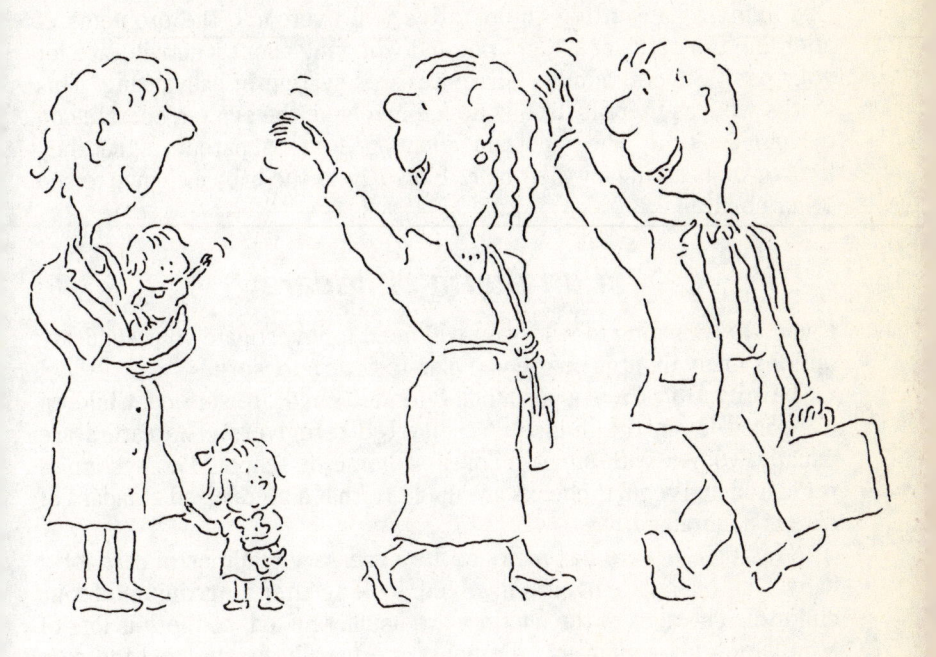

One of the greatest survival techniques for parents is to have time out from their baby. This is not a luxury but a necessity if you are to maintain the quality of your care-giving. Your baby will benefit from having time with other people, as they provide different experiences and activities. Being cared for by others also helps your baby develop trust in you returning after a short period of separation, and you will usually feel mentally refreshed and pleased to be reunited with your baby.

At first it may be very difficult to leave your baby for even short periods of time. Partners, grandparents or close friends are usually the best form of childcare to start with, as you will feel confident that your baby is in a loving environment while you are away.

SPECIAL SITUATIONS

Occasional care

In many communities there are occasional care centres for babies and small children. This minding service is usually offered at minimal cost to the parents, and there may be a restriction on the number of hours of care per child per month. Many parents use this time for shopping or taking part in some regular group activity.

Joining a babysitting co-operative will overcome the problems of affording the occasional night out and worrying about who will care for your baby. Several families share a roster system of babysitting. This works well, as there is usually no fee involved; the system operates on exchange of time. The important advantage for most parents is that they know who is caring for their baby. It also gives the baby a chance to see other children.

Long-term childcare

If you are returning to work you will need to investigate your childcare options many months before you plan to return to work.

Family Day Care is a council-operated childcare service. Children are cared for in the homes of registered caregivers. The carers are usually women with small children at home or school. The system is regulated and regular checks are made so that a recognised standard of care is maintained.

This type of care has many of the necessary qualities of care for a baby. One main caregiver is involved, looking after a maximum of four children. The ages of the children are usually mixed, so there is lots of stimulation for your baby. The hours are usually flexible and the cost reasonable.

Long day care centres are either government funded or privately operated, and the fees vary enormously. Subsidies are available at the government-operated centres and are worth asking about if you are a lone parent or a low-income family.

In many areas there are long waiting lists for childcare places. Start to plan well in advance if you are considering the need for regular childcare; you can always cancel or postpone your booking if you change your mind.

How do I choose childcare?

There are many types of childcare, so it is important that you choose the type that fulfils your basic needs. Aspects you may have to consider are religion, locality, cost, the educational experiences offered to the children and the general atmosphere of the centre.

When visiting childcare centres, take along a checklist of the qualities you wish to consider so that you can answer the following questions:

1. **Safety and hygiene:** Are the equipment and toys in good repair? Is there childproof fencing around the perimeter of the property? Are there grassed play areas? Are there adequate handwashing facilities? Are the nappy changing areas isolated from the food and bottle preparation areas?

2. **Qualifications the be staff:** Do the staff have teaching and/or childcare qualifications? Is there someone on duty at all times who has a current first aid certificate or nursing qualifications?

3. **Ratio of staff to children:** This is dependent on government regulations and can be checked through your local council or Family and Community Services office. The usual ratio is one carer for every four children.

4. **Daily programme:** Is there a general daily routine, including regular periods of regular periods of sleep time? Is there a variety of activities available from energetic to quiet?

5. **Meals:** Do you bring your baby's meals, or are they supplied? Are special diets taken into account if necessary? Are the meals offered nutritionally well balanced?

6. **Attitudes to parents:** Are you made to feel welcome and invited to involve yourself in the centre's activities? Are you encouraged to ring and check if your baby has settled? Can you visit at any time? What happens if you are running late and cannot pick up your baby on time?

7. **Attitudes to children:** What methods of discipline are used? Are crying children being attended to by the staff? Do the children look happy? Do the staff look happy? Does the supervision of children appear adequate?

8. The most important question to ask yourself is, **do you feel happy about leaving your child at the centre?** If you are uneasy about safety standards or the personalities of the staff caring for your baby, you may spend most of the time your child is in care worrying. Childcare should free you, physically and emotionally, from the cares of looking after your child, so that you can get on with the other things in your life for a while.

SPECIAL SITUATIONS

Returning to work

Many women are choosing to return to work within the first year of their babies' lives, or are forced to for financial reasons. There will be many issues to think about and discuss with your partner if you are considering returning to work.

Who will care for our baby?

Often the ideal person to replace the parent's care for a small baby is a grandparent, but this is not always possible. Childcare needs to be organised early, as vacancies at childcare centres can be difficult to find. It is worthwhile placing your baby's name on a waiting list at least a year in advance of your anticipated return to work. You may feel happier on your first day back at work if you have left your baby at the centre for short periods in the preceding weeks, so that she has become familiar with her new carers.

Can I negotiate shorter working hours?

Employers will sometimes allow you part-time work, with the hours gradually increasing until you have settled into your new routine. This option is worth investigating. Check with your union, as there may be an award requirement covering the return to work after maternity leave, which will support you in your request for shorter working hours.

What happens if our baby is unwell?

Which parent will stay home and care for her, or will both parents share the responsibility? Is there a neighbour, relative or friend who can act as a back-up person and who is prepared to care for your baby in an emergency, or for short periods of time?

How will the family manage the increased workload?

It is wise to discuss the division of household chores with your partner before you return to work, as it will be impossible to combine a full-time job with the already heavy workload of a housekeeper, cook and mother. Partners need to be realistic about what they are prepared to do to assist with the general running of the house and looking after children. If the workload is too great for both of you to cope with, look at ways you can adjust the household budget so that you can afford a house-cleaning service. Take short cuts with your housework, and do only the chores that you consider to be necessary for safety or hygiene. It is easy to skip meals or fall into poor eating habits when you are extremely busy or tired. Cook double quantities of weekend meals; these can be frozen for the following week, when you are too tired to prepare a meal.

How will our family life be affected?

It is important to make sure that you have time together as a family. Many families are so busy working that they forget to enjoy sharing each other's company. If you cannot see much of each other during the week, make sure you spend time together on the weekend.

When will we get time out?

It is easy to neglect your own wellbeing for the sake of the family. Make sure each of you has time to her or himself, in which to relax, pursue interests outside the home and fulfil personal needs.

What if things don't work out?

Feelings of guilt are common for working parents; many women, in particular, have mixed feelings about returning to work. The important things for small children are that they have a stable home base and that the basic care they receive at the childcare centre is consistent with the care they receive at home. If, after several weeks of working, your feelings of guilt are still worrying you, examine the causes of your concern. Are your childcare arrangements a problem? Has your baby's behaviour altered for the worse, or does she seem unhappy? Are you finding the emotional and/or physical effects of working difficult to cope with? Is it possible for your partner to stay at home while you work? Alternatives to working outside your home can be explored; many people are able to work from home, which enables them to care for their children while earning some money. Explore the need for childcare in your area; you may be able to care for other children in your home.

Will I continue to breastfeed my baby?

If you are enjoying breastfeeding, there is no reason to wean. See page 137 for ways of combining work and breastfeeding, and consider methods of partially breastfeeding.

All mothers are working mothers. Some are able to make choices about staying home with their children or going out to work. Many mothers would prefer to stay with their children, but are forced into working away from their children for financial reasons. Whatever their situation, all women need access to childcare so that they can have time to attend to their own physical and emotional needs. Children thrive on quality time

SPECIAL SITUATIONS

with their parents; how you spend the limited time you have with your children is more important than the sum total of hours you have together. Leave reading the paper and watching television until your children are in bed; read them stories at bedtime; play with them while they are having their baths, and generally enjoy their company. Preparing and freezing food ahead of time will leave you extra time to spend with your children in the evenings.

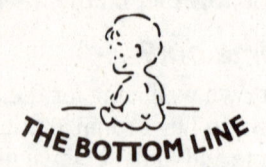

THE BOTTOM LINE

- Use occasional care in the early months to obtain time for yourself.
- Plan well ahead if you are going to need family day care or long day care.
- Visit the childcare centre you are considering and assess it for yourself. If you feel comfortable there, chances are your child will be happy there too.
- Know ahead of time what will be done if you cannot pick up your child, or if your child falls ill.
- Negotiate with your partner the sharing of the household workload.

Appendices

APPENDIX I

Safety

Making sure your home is safe will be one of the most continuous and important tasks you will perform as a parent. You need to become alert to potential dangers, both inside and outside your home. This will mean being alert on visits to relatives' and friends' houses, as well as on shopping trips and outings to parks and playgrounds.

The first aid kit

Kits can be bought from first aid associations, chemists or hardware stores, or you can make your own. Make sure it is in a container that is dust proof and easy to carry. Your first aid kit should contain the following items.

- tweezers
- scissors
- thermometer
- **paracetamol for infants and children**
- Syrup of Ipecac — Check the expiry date regularly and replace it if it is out of date. Do not administer without medical advice.
- calamine lotion
- antiseptic solution
- medicine glass or measurer
- sterile crepe bandages
- sterile gauze bandages
- adhesive dressings of various sizes
- adhesive plaster
- safety pins
- roll of cotton wool
- triangular bandage for—sling this can be made from a square of old sheeting (90 cm—3 feet square)
- plastic bags with sealable tops to carry water in, or for making ice packs. Alternatively, re-usable hot and cold packs are available from your chemist.

SAFETY

Keep emergency numbers handy—put a list by the phone and keep it up to date. Fill in and photocopy the list on page 14 of this book for ready referenee

Childproofing your home

It is never too early to childproof your house. You certainly should do it before your baby starts to crawl. Each room should be systematically checked for potential hazards.

It is now possible to get **circuit breakers** for electrical outlets. These will lower the risk of accident and improve your peace of mind. The installation of **smoke detectors** will alert you to a fire. These devices save many lives each year.

It is possible to get **locks for drawers and cupboards** from a hardware store or from the safety centre at some hospitals. Such centres carry a large array of goods, including **curly cords** for electrical appliances, medicine cupboards, safety plugs for power points and child resistant taps.

Try to **remove most hazards** and be consistent with the rules regarding the hazards you cannot remove. Set limits early and follow them through. Try not to make too many rules or restrictions, as you will have to continually enforce them until your child is three years old or more. You will have to continue checking for hazards around the home even after this time, of course, but you will have developed good habits both for your baby and for yourself.

Sometimes avoiding hazards calls for a little creativity. **Playpens**, for example, are a good place for you *or* the baby when you are doing the ironing. That is, you can either place the baby inside the playpen, or place the pen against the wall where the power point is and put yourself and the ironing board inside, allowing the baby to crawl around on the floor outside. Put a table nearby for your ironed clothes if you are ironing inside the playpen, so that you need not move from the playpen until you are ready to finish.

Keep a watchful eye out for **danger areas** (kitchens, bathrooms, laundries and garages are usually full of hazards) and remember that children do not have the same awareness of danger as adults, and often are not physically capable of avoiding danger.

Always **check where your baby is before you answer the phone**, and if necessary bring the baby with you. This is not always an ideal arrangement, but you may be longer on the phone than you expected, and accidents can occur very quickly.

Kitchen

Buy **catches and childproof locks** for your cupboards and drawers. Place **knives and scissors** in a high cupboard or drawer. Move knives attached to walls in sheaths to a safer position as children are good climbers.

Place **detergents and dishwashing liquid** in a high cupboard. **Dishwasher powder** is highly poisonous and easily accessible to children in the doors of dishwashers. Always close and fasten the catch of the dishwasher door if you are leaving powder in it.

Take care if you are using a **microwave** to heat food, as there is a risk of overheating. There have been several cases of babies' mouths being severely burned by microwaved formulas and foods.

Do not allow the **cords of electrical equipment** such as the frying pan, toaster or jug to hang within reach of your baby. **Curly cords** are now available for electrical equipment, and if your budget allows it, buy cordless articles like jugs.

Turn all **saucepan handles** towards the back or centre of the stove when you are cooking, so that children cannot grab them and pull them down onto themselves. **Stove guards** are now available to prevent saucepans being pulled from the top of the stove. Replace matches for gas stoves with an automatic lighter, and keep it out of the reach of your baby.

Wipe up spills on the floor as soon as they occur to minimise the risk of slipping.

There is a very real risk of **burns and scalds** from the hot glass of the oven doors, from oven plates, boiled water for formula preparation, coffee, tea and other hot liquids. Do not carry or nurse your baby when you are drinking hot fluids, and do not cook with your baby in your arms or a carry pouch.

Children can sometimes climb onto open **oven doors** and make the oven topple over, so be sure you always close the door and discourage your child from touching it.

Replace tablecloths with placemats when your baby is small, so that he cannot pull any heavy or breakable objects, cutlery, hot liquids or plates of food onto himself. Take care where you place his highchair or stroller, especially when near tables, as he may pull hot food or liquids towards him and spill them on himself. Keep hot dishes in the middle of the table.

Leave one cupboard containing plastic articles free of childproof catches. When your child is older, he can have a special cupboard, so that the entire kitchen is not out of bounds to him.

A **barrier** at the kitchen door, or a **playpen** set up where you can keep an eye on it, is a good idea if you are cooking. This allows your baby to see you but keeps him out from under your feet.

Have a **fire extinguisher** and a **fire blanket** handy.

Bathroom

Children should not be left alone in the bathroom at any age. They can easily slip over, and can drown even in the water in the toilet bowl. When the bathroom is not in use, keep the door closed.

Take care that you do not slip on the bathroom floor. If it is wet, put down a **bathmat** to lessen the risk of falls. **Non-slip mats or strips in the bath** also help prevent accidents.

Medicines in unlocked cupboards are a hazard. When tablets and medicines are no longer needed, they should be put down the toilet (all except antibiotics, which can contaminate the water system), burned in the incinerator, or returned to your local chemist for safe disposal. Do not put them in the garbage bin, where they could be found and consumed by children. Buy a safety cupboard, available from safety centres and some hardware stores, for the medicines that you are currently using. If you have medicines that need refrigeration, place them at the back of the fridge out of children's reach.

Hot water taps present a risk of scalds; 90 per cent of hot tap burns occur in the bathroom. Make a habit of running the hot and cold water together, then running a small amount of cold water again to cool the tap. This will be a good habit for when your baby gets older, as it prevents him burning himself if he touches the tap. Test the temperature of the water on the inside of your forearm, as this is a more sensitive area than either your hands or your elbows. The installation of a **temperature controlling device,** for example a tempering valve or a thermostatic mixing valve, is the most efficient method. These devices need to be installed by a plumber.

Electrical appliances and water can be a fatal combination. Wall-mounted heaters are safer than floor heaters for the bathroom. Remove hairdryers and razors from the bathroom for safety, even if this is not very convenient.

Dining and living areas

There will be objects in the dining and living areas that cannot be moved out of your child's reach; these will probably include the **television, video and stereo** units. You and your partner will have to decide what your baby may not touch, and be firm and consistent in keeping him away until he is about three years old. Although children learn very quickly, they will still try to do things you have told them not to, to make sure that you are serious. If you are not careful you could end up saying 'no' far more often than you would like.

It is sometimes easier and better for both you and your baby if you **put away very precious, irreplaceable or fragile items**. Even removing ornaments and other items such as compact disc, record and tape collections to a higher position will not protect them once your baby is climbing, which will be from about ten months in some children.

Cabinets containing **glass and china**, and drawers containing **cutlery**, should either be locked or put on your list of untouchables. **Bookcases** should be anchored to the wall if possible, to prevent them falling on the climbing child. Table lamps and other potentially dangerous items, such as large vases and glass objects, fish bowls and plants should be moved out of your baby's reach, or you should forbid him to touch them.

Fish tanks can be fascinating for small children. Make sure that they are stable and that your child cannot climb up and reach the water. Take care that there is no electrical equipment nearby that your baby could drop into the water.

Alcohol should be placed out of children's reach or locked away.

Extreme care should be taken when your child is in the same room as an **open fire or a heater**. A fire guard should be used at all times, and vigilant supervision is also necessary. Dress your baby in non-flammable clothing.

Keep an eye on your baby when he is around **tables with square corners**, especially coffee tables, as he can easily fall onto such corners or bump his head as he tries to pull himself up into a standing position. Table-corner protectors are available at hardware stores and safety centres.

Highchairs should have a wide base and a safety strap that goes both around your baby's waist and up between his legs. Check the hinges and catches for protruding screws, and make sure that they close properly.

If you have glass doors or floor-to-ceiling windows, place stickers or tape at your child's eye level to prevent him running headlong into the glass. You will have to move the markers up as your child grows.

Bedroom

Bedside lamps can be pulled over on top of your baby, causing injury and a fire risk. Do not cover the bedside lamp with a nappy or other material to dim the light; this presents a fire hazard. Use a night light or dimmer switch.

The **corners of beds and bedside tables** can also have sharp corners capable of causing injury, so watch your baby when he is near these, or put corner-protectors on them.

The **dressing-table** should be clear of medications, perfumes, small coins and other small objects your baby could swallow.

If you own a **water bed**, do not leave your baby on it, as the risk of him smothering is high.

Nursery

Safety measures to take in the nursery have been mentioned throughout this book. See the section on setting up the nursery (pages 23–6) and using a cot (page 104).

Laundry

Laundries are usually full of potential hazards. It is best to keep the door closed unless you are using the room. The risk of your children falling from or into the **washing machine** is a real one, once they have started to climb.

If you live in a flat or unit, or have a carport, and you use the laundry to store items normally kept in the garage, read the section on **garage safety**.

Washing liquid, bleach, oven cleaners, corrosive poisons such as drain cleaners, and cleaning fluids should be put out of reach of children, and the lids and caps of containers should be screwed or pressed on firmly.

Buckets should be emptied immediately after use and turned upside down to reduce the risk of drowning. Care should also be taken with buckets of nappy sterilising liquid for the same reason; these require a secure lid. Small children can drown in 40 centimetres (16 inches) of water.

If storing **plastic bags** for future use, make sure they are out of reach of children.

Toys

Toys for children should be appropriate for their age and should be thoroughly checked for safety and regularly inspected for damage. They should be **non-flammable and non-toxic**, and preferably easy to wash. Plastic packaging is potentially dangerous, and should be disposed of immediately to prevent suffocation.

Small buttons and eyes on teddies and dolls, and beads and small batteries, can all be swallowed by babies and toddlers; make sure your baby cannot remove them. **Sharp objects** and **brittle plastic toys** are a hazard. **Heavy toys** should be avoided, and **wooden toys** checked for splinters. **Seams on stuffed toys** should be checked regularly. **Walking trolleys** should be stable and well balanced.

Toy boxes can be climbed both on and into, and care should be taken with heavy lids, as these can fall on small heads, fingers and limbs. Hinges can also pinch. It may be easier to remove the lid and hinges while the baby is small. If your child's toy box is large enough for him to get inside, it should have air holes on all four sides. Small children can also climb onto and fall off **rocking horses and other movable toys**, so find a safe way to immobilise these toys unless you are with your child to supervise him.

Clothing

All your child's clothing should be fire resistant; look at the compulsory labels when you buy clothing or when it is given to you. There are three levels: low fire danger, styled to reduce fire and high fire danger.

Bodysuits with tight feet can restrict the circulation; this can become a problem as some garments shrink with washing. They can also cause your baby to trip or slip once he is crawling and pulling himself up into a standing position.

Mittens and bootees can also be dangerous if tied too tight. Check the ties and place your finger inside the tie to check for tightness; it should slide inside easily. Check to see that there are no loose threads on the inside that could wrap around your baby's fingers or toes.

Unless it is very cold, crawling and toddling children are safer left **barefooted inside the house**. When walking outside, they should have well-fitting shoes with flexible soles to give them good grip and a sole thick enough to prevent cuts from broken glass and other sharp objects.

A **dummy** can be pinned to your child's clothing with a safety pin and a short piece of ribbon when you are taking him out, but you should not pin his dummy to his clothing when at home. If your child is crawling and active, the dummy will drag on the floor. The rubber on dummies tends to become brittle as they get older, and can be bitten off by older children. Regular checks and replacement can reduce the risk of your child inhaling the broken piece. Do not put your baby's dummy in your mouth to clean it before giving it to him; this only adds more bacteria to it. Have three dummies and always have a sterile one handy if he drops one on the ground.

SAFETY

Falls

Falls can occur at any age. Small babies can fall from beds, lounges, change tables and carry baskets. Develop good practices for avoiding falls in the early months of your child's life, and these will soon become habits for the years ahead.

Ensure that you have a **strap on your change table** and that you do not leave your baby unattended on the table at any time. This may mean that you have to carry your baby with you or put him on the floor if you have forgotten something or you need to answer the door or the phone. Do not prop your baby in the corner of the lounge, as he can work his way to the edge and fall off.

Straps should always be used to hold your baby firmly in his stroller, pram, bouncinette or highchair. His **highchair** should have a wide base, so that it cannot overbalance.

Take care when **carrying your baby** that you support his head with the crook of your arm. As well as being more comfortable for your baby, this ensures that his head does not hit door frames or other objects that you pass. **Carry baskets** are safer with the handles tied together, so that if one handle slips from your grasp, your baby's weight does not unbalance the basket.

Bouncinettes should only be placed on the floor, and not on benches, tables or bed, as they can move as the baby bounces.

The **catches** on all equipment for children, including prams, strollers, highchairs and playpens, should be checked regularly to ensure that they cannot pinch or cut their small hands.

The **brake** on your baby's pram or stroller should always be applied when you are parking it on an incline.

Staircases should be blocked with barriers at both top and bottom so that crawling babies and small children do not fall. If you are making your own gates, make sure that the distance beteween the rungs is no less than 5 cm (2") and no wider than 8.5 cm ($3\frac{1}{2}$"), so that small heads and limbs cannot be caught between them.

Make sure your **furniture** is stable before your baby learns to pull himself into a standing position at about nine months of age.

Take care if you have a **balcony** or if you visit someone with a balcony. Ensure that the door to the balcony is closed or blocked, and if you are out on the balcony keep your child away from plant stands and other objects that could be used for climbing.

Firearms

The decision to keep a firearm on the property should not be made lightly, as many accidents occur every year involving both children and adults and firearms.

Firearms should be kept in a high, locked cupboard, and the key should be kept in a separate place, out of the reach of children, and preferably somewhere where they are either forbidden or very unlikely to go. **Pistols** should be stored in personal safes, as instructed by the licence requirements.

Ammunition should be stored away from the firearm, also in a locked cupboard. The firearm should be stored unloaded and with the bolt removed if it is a bolt-action rifle. The firearm should be **loaded and cleaned** away from children.

Childproofing around your home

Garage

Go through your garage and place all **potentially lethal substances** well out of reach of children. Many garages contain poisons, weed-killers, turpentine, paint, lawnmower petrol and pool chemicals, to name just a few dangerous substances.

All **tools and garden implements**, including the lawnmower, should be locked away from your children. Unplug all **electrical work equipment** not in use, and place it out of your children's reach.

When **storing objects** in the garage, make sure that they cannot fall from the position in which you have placed them. Do not store liquids, powders or pastes in soft drink bottles or food containers in which they may be mistaken for food and consumed.

If you have an **old fridge** in the garage or yard, or a similar piece of equipment that a child could lock himself in by accident, either get rid of it or remove the lock to make it safe.

Water safety

Drowning is a common cause of death of children in Australia. It is important, when your child is near any body of water, to **keep a close eye on him**.

If you have a **swimming pool**, you should have an approved **safety fence** around it, and **safety catches** on the gate. Be very strict about supervision both of your own child and visitors' children. Safety fences and catches are not legally required in all states of Australia yet, so be sure, even if you have fenced your own pool, that your neighbours' pool is not a potential hazard for your children.

When unused, the pool should be **covered**. Even small inflatable

SAFETY

swimming pools can be dangerous. These should be emptied and turned upside down when not in use; as well as the potential for drowning, there is a danger of the water becoming contaminated.

Pool chemicals should be stored in a locked area. **Pool filters** are also potentially lethal to small children; always check that you have closed the lid properly.

Children should be given **swimming lessons** and taught **pool safety**. It is possible to teach children under two years to float, but not to swim. It is important to remember that swimming or water safety classes give children confidence in the water but will not prevent them from drowning. Children can hit their heads on the edge of the pool as they fall in, and no amount of swimming classes will assist if they are unconscious. Keeping a close watch on them during all water play is the only way to guarantee their safety.

Water tanks are a potential source of danger for older children. As children grow older they become better and more adventurous at climbing, and can fall into or off a water tank. **Local creeks, rivers** and other pools of water such as garden fountains are potential hazards for children of any age once they are mobile. If you have a **fish pond** in your garden, cover it with strong mesh to prevent babies and toddlers falling in the water.

The best means of preventing water-related accidents is supervision by an adult. Older children are usually too busy enjoying themselves to supervise properly and making them responsible for small children's lives is asking too much of them. Even the most sensible child cannot see potential dangers as easily as adults.

Outdoor play equipment

Outdoor play equipment should be **sturdy and safe** with **soft sand areas** underneath to prevent injury. Check regularly for the presence of **spiders** in these areas, and if you live in a bush area be aware of the dangers of **snakes and ticks**. (See page 257 for treatment.)

Make sure the equipment is appropriate for the age of the child. The most common accidents related to the use of swings are falls and children being hit by swings. Keep a keen eye on children playing on the equipment.

When sandpits are not in use, keep them covered to prevent them being fouled by animals and check for spiders prior to re-use.

Gardening

When you are gardening, be careful that your **tools** do not fall into your

APPENDICES

children's hands and keep your children away from **chemicals and lawn foods**. A large locked trunk is a good storage place for all these dangerous things.

When you are **mowing the lawn**, small babies and children should stay inside the house so that they cannot be injured by flying stones or twigs. When you have finished, replace the lawnmower in the garage straight away, to reduce the risk of your children cutting themselves on the blades.

Be sure that the **garden gates** are closed and secured if you are working in the garden with your child. It only takes a moment's distraction on your part to lose sight of your child, and in that time he can escape onto the road.

Be aware of the dangers present in your garden from **poisonous plants**. Some common plants such as azaleas and oleanders are poisonous, and it is not wise to grow these in your garden while you have young children. A handbook on poisonous plants can be obtained from the health department in your state.

You should also be aware of the types of **venomous spiders and snakes** that are common in your area. Funnel-web and red-back spiders are common in certain areas of Australia, and you should be able to recognise the spiders themselves and their likely habitats. When you are moving wood from a woodpile, keep children away, wear heavy gloves and do not put your hand into any area that you cannot see. Ticks are also dangerous to children; if you visit or live in a bush area, you should check your baby and yourself when you return home. See pages 256–7 for the treatment of snake and insect bites.

The fire danger presented by **barbecues** and **incinerators** should never be ignored. Children are usually fascinated by fire and you should supervise them carefully. They should not wear flowing articles of clothing such as dressing gowns or nighties around a fire, but should be dressed in close-fitting clothing, such as a tracksuit. Never light any fire using flammable liquid; this is extremely dangerous for you and sets a bad example for your children.

Sunburn

Babies of less than twelve months should be kept out of the sun as much as possible, especially between 10 a.m. and 2 p.m. in the summer months (11 a.m and 3 p.m. if your state has daylight saving). Obviously it is not possible to keep your child completely out of the sun, as sometimes you will need to do such things as shopping that involves going outside in the

SAFETY

middle of the day. At these times your baby should be protected with a **sun protection factor 15 plus, broad spectrum and water resistant sunscreen**. The sunscreen should be applied twenty minutes before going outside and reapplied every two hours.

Babies should be covered with a cotton sheet or with cool clothing that has long sleeves and long legs, even when in the car or pram. Remember that sun also burns when it is reflected off sand and water.

Put a **sunhat** on your baby; this should have elastic or be tied on, as a small child will usually try to remove it as soon as it is placed on his head. Be persistent and keep replacing the hat, and your baby will soon give up. Cotton hats are best in very hot regions.

Set a good example; make wearing a hat and applying sunscreen part of the ritual before any family member goes outside.

If you live in a very hot region, try to find **a shady place to put your baby** when he is outside, but be careful that he is not exposed to filtered sunlight. Make sure he is taking **adequate fluids** if you need to be out for any length of time, as babies are very prone to dehydration. Water is the best drink for small babies, as long as it is boiled. If you live in an area with a fluoridated water supply, the water has the added advantage of being good for your baby's teeth.

Take care when you are travelling **in the car**, as your baby can be burnt through the windows. Use a screen fitted to your car window to protect your baby. Do not hang a nappy, towel or other cloth across the window as this will obstruct the driver's view.

In the car

Always place your baby in **an approved car safety capsule or seat** when taking him anywhere in the car. Your state road and traffic authority will answer any questions about the purchase, rental or installation of capsules or seats. You can rent them from local hospitals, councils, community service groups and some private organisations. If you have a station wagon or hatchback, you will need to buy an extension strap to fit the capsule or seat properly.

If you are borrowing or buying a **secondhand capsule**, make sure that it has not been in an accident. If it has any cracks, frayed straps or damaged buckles, do not use it.

The **capsule liner** you use should be the one provided by the manufacturer, as it is designed not to allow the baby to slide out of the capsule on impact. Although home-made or bought liners sometimes look more attractive, they are not as safe.

APPENDICES

Do not place your baby in the capsule with a cuddly or blanket wrapped round him. Strap him in and then tuck the cuddly in around him. A wrapped baby is much more likely to slide out of the capsule in the event of an accident. Check the safety strap at regular intervals, and remove any lint or fluff that has accumulated, so that the fastener can grip properly. Some brands have a harness. The shoulder straps should be level with or above the baby's shoulders. You need to adjust the crotch strap first.

Once your baby can hold his head up well (at about six months), he can be placed in a recommended and approved **car seat** when travelling. Remember to reposition your car window sun screen to protect your baby. Do not restrict your vision while driving by hanging nappies or towels from the window to shade your baby.

Car seats can get uncomfortably hot in the sun; cover with a cloth while you are away from the car.

Children should not be left unattended in cars at ANY time. It may be difficult to follow this advice, especially if you have more than one child, but it is essential that you do. Children dehydrate quickly in closed cars, and toddlers can let off handbrakes or play with cigarette lighters.

Make a habit of **never leaving the keys in the ignition** of the car; this keeps them away from toddlers and also prevents you being locked out with your child in the car. Carry a second set of keys just in case.

The car should not be used as a place for children to play. When not in use, it should be locked and parked in a garage, if available.

Newer cars are fitted with **childproof locks** on the rear doors; make sure these are in the 'lock' position before you drive off anywhere. **When getting babies and children out of the car, do so on the kerb side** of the car, and be careful in shopping centre car parks where this is not possible.

Do a head count before backing out of your driveway. Make sure you know where your children and the neighbour's children are before you drive off.

Teach children not to sit or play behind the car, even when it is not in use.

Animals

When your baby is new, your **dog** may become jealous of him because you seem to be giving him all your attention. See page 53 for ways of dealing with your dog's jealousy.

SAFETY

Cats like to curl up next to a baby in a bassinette, and your cat could possibly smother your baby by doing this. It is better to shut your baby's bedroom door (and the window, if you do not have screens) when he is sleeping if your cat normally lives in the house.

Wash your hands well after handling any animals, and keep pets healthy by immunisation and regular worming and de-fleaing. **Feed pets** somewhere where your baby cannot disturb them, and do not allow your child to play near their feed bowls or bedding, or with their toys. **Discourage your child** from patting or picking up dogs or cats that you do not know, and wash his hands after he has patted any animal.

Even with an animal that you do know and trust, **keep a close watch** on your child and be prepared to intervene quickly if either looks like hurting the other. Children can be very cruel to animals without knowing what they are doing, and a cat or dog pushed to its limit will scratch or snap with very little warning. If you watch, you will be aware of any dangerous situation developing; remove your child before he comes to any harm or hurts the animal.

Away from home

Prevention is better than cure, and people whom you visit, particularly people who do not have children, may not be as safety conscious as yourself. When you are out visiting, have a quick look around for danger spots on arrival. Most people you visit will be happy to help you make the area safer by moving breakable objects, closing doors or blocking off areas.

Older friends and relatives may keep their medications beside their beds or on the kitchen table. Medications can be very attractive to small children, as they sometimes look like sweets. Your friends or relatives will not mind moving them to a safer place while your children are there.

Do not leave your baby alone at any time when you are out. There is a risk of animals or persons taking the baby if, for example, you leave him outside a shop in his stroller.

APPENDICES

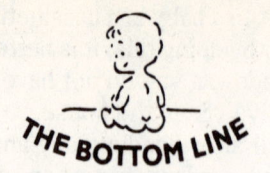

THE BOTTOM LINE

- Plan ahead; childproof your house before your child is mobile.
- Try to stay one step ahead of your child's development, so that when he decides, for example, to start pulling himself up on the furniture, you will already have removed or secured all unstable chairs and tables.
- Know the danger areas in any place your baby plays in, and know where he is at all times.
- Be prepared for accidents; learn resuscitation techniques and first aid, and have emergency telephone numbers handy for when you need help in a hurry.

APPENDIX II

Support services — Australia and New Zealand

The following list is not comprehensive; there are now many services parents can utilise to gain support and information. Your early childhood health nurse, the community health centre, the local council or the library are your best contacts for discovering the services available to you.

In most cases, only the head office of the organisation has been listed. Staff will direct you to the branch closest to your home.

All Australian telephone numbers will contain 8 digits in the next few years. These changes will be implementd as follows:

	Area code	Change
May 1996	089	change area code to 08 and add 89 to beginning of existing number
July 1996	02	add 9 to beginning of existing number
August 1996	08	add 8 to beginning of existing number
August 1996	002	change area code to 03 and add 62 to beginning of existing number
May 1997	09	change area code to 08 and add 9 to beginning of existing number
August 1997	06	change area code to 02 and add 62 to beginning of existing number

APPENDICES

24-HOUR PHONE ADVISORY/ COUNSELLING SERVICE

Tresillian Family Care Centre
(02) 569 5400
1800 637 357 free call outside Sydney metropolitan area

Royal Plunket Society (Inc.)
96 Symonds Street
Auckland NZ
(09) 377 4365
0800 10 1067 (24-hour toll-free Helpline)

Plunket Karitane Family Centres
159 Landscape Road
Mt Eden Auckland NZ
(09) 620 8539
0800 10 1067 (24-hour free child health service)

RESIDENTIAL PARENTCRAFT HOSPITALS

These services provide 24-hour phone counselling.

Tresillian Family Care Centre
2 Shaw Street
Petersham NSW 2049
(02) 568 3633

Tresillian Family Care Centre
2 Second Avenue
Willoughby NSW 2068
(02) 9958 8931

Tresillian Family Care Centre
1B Barber Avenue
Kingswood NSW 2747
(047) 24 2124

Tresillian Outreach Domiciliary Service
Wollstonecraft (02) 436 4086

Petersham (02) 560 0777
Tresillian Day Stay Clinics
Petersham (02) 560 0777
Wollstonecraft (02) 436 4086
Penrith (047) 24 2124

Karitane Mothercraft Society
Cnr Horsley Drive & Mitchell Street
Fairfield NSW 2163
(02) 794 1800

O'Connell Family Centre
(formerly The Gray Sisters)
6 Mont Albert Road
Canterbury Vic 3126
(03) 9882 2327

Queen Elizabeth Centre
56 Lytton Street
Carlton Vic 3053
(03) 9347 2777

Tweedle Baby Hospital
398 Barkly Street
Footscray Vic 3011
(03) 9689 1577

Riverton Centre
75 Christian Street
Clayfield Qld 4011
(07) 3862 2333

St Pauls Terrace Day Stay Riverton Centre
184 St Paul's Terrace
Fortitude Valley Qld 4006
(07) 252 8555

Child, Adolescent and Family Health Service
Torrens House Mothercraft Hospital
295 South Terrace
Adelaide SA 5000
(08) 236 0400
(008) 18 8082 (24-hour phone counselling)

Ngala Family Resource Centre
9 George Street
Kensington WA 6151
(09) 333 9777
After Hours Hotline: (09) 367 3256

Parenting Centre
(day stay only)
232 Newtown Rd
Tas 7008
(002) 33 2700
1 800 808 178 (24-hour Parent Information Telephone Assistance Service)

Queen Elizabeth II Home
Alinga Street
Canberra City ACT 2601
(06) 248 0813

There are no residential services in the Northern Territory or New Zealand, but support is available from the following services:

Royal Darwin Hospital
Rocklands Drive
Tiwi NT 0810
(089) 22 8888

SUPPORT SERVICES — AUSTRALIA AND NEW ZEALAND

Alice Springs Hospital
Gap Road
Alice Springs NT 0870
(089) 51 7777

Royal New Zealand
  Plunket Society (Inc.)
96 Symonds Street
Auckland 1 NZ
(09) 377 4365
(0800) 101 067 (24-hour
  Helpline)

Plunket Karitane Family
  Support Unit
159 Landscape Road
Mt Eden Auckland NZ
(09) 620 8539

Plunket Karitane Family
  Centre
77 Constable Street
Newtown NZ
(04) 389 6075

Plunket Karitane Family
  Support Unit
2 David Street
Dunedin North NZ
(03) 477 9257
(03) 389 5588

Plunket Karitane Family
  Support Unit
333 Riccarton Road
Christchurch NZ
(03) 348 9447

**POST-NATAL
DEPRESSION SUPPORT
AND/OR TREATMENT
GROUPS**
All of the residential
services listed above are
involved in the treatment
and support of families with
post-natal depression.
Other post-natal
depression support groups
include the following:

Postnatal Depression
  Support Group (ACT) Inc.
PO Box 1705
Tuggeranong Mail Centre
  ACT 2901
(06) 291 0418 Kim
  (Telephone Support)
(06) 237 5108 Janet
  (Current President)

Victoria
(03) 9758 4053
(Not a support group, but
refers people on and offers
counselling and literature to
people suffering with PND.)

Queensland
(07) 209 2773

Helen Mayo House
Glenside Hospital
PO Box 17
Eastwood SA 5063
Postnatal Residential Unit
  catering for families with
  children 0–5 years
24-hour Telephone Support
  Service
(08) 303 1183 or (08) 303
  1425

**BREASTFEEDING
ADVICE**
See also 'Residential
  Parentcraft Hospitals'.

Tresillian Family Care
  Centres
(24-hour phone advisory/
  counselling service NSW)
(02) 569 5400
1800 637 357

Walker House
  Family Health Centre
17A Walkers Avenue
Newnham Tas 7248
(003) 266 188
(008) 808 178 (after hours)

Nursing Mothers
  Association of Australia:
NSW   (02) 686 4141
Vic   (03) 9878 3304
Qld   (07) 266 3119
SA   (08) 339 6783
WA   (09) 309 5393
Tas   (002) 29 5461
NT   (089) 27 5957
ACT   (06) 258 8928

La Leche League New
  Zealand, Inc.
PO Box 13-383
Wellington NZ
(04) 478 1315

**CONTRACEPTIVE
ADVICE
Family Planning
Association**
This association will advise
you with regard to your
contraceptive needs, and
also offers advice,
counselling and referral for
pregnancy, breast
problems, women's health
and sexual problems:

Family Planning Association
328-336 Liverpool Road
Ashfield NSW 2131
(02) 716 6566

Family Planning Association
266-270 Church Street
Richmond Vic 3121
(03) 9429 1177

APPENDICES

Family Planning Association (Sexual Counselling & Sexual Health Screening)
100 Alfred Street
Fortitude Valley
Qld 4006
(07) 3252 5151

Family Planning Assocation
17 Phillips Street
Kensington SA 5068
(08) 31 5177

Family Planning Association
70 Roe Street
Northbridge WA 6000
(09) 227 6177

Family Planning Association
73 Federal Street
North Hobart Tas 7000
(002) 34 7200

Shop 11 Rapid Creek Shopping Centre
Trower Road
Rapid Creek NT 0210
(089) 48 0144

Health Promotion Centre
Childers Street
Canberra ACT 2600
(06) 247 3077

Family Planning Association
Health Promotion Centre
Administration/Education/ Resource Unit
2nd Floor,
30 Ponsonby Road
Newton Auckland NZ
(09) 360 0360

Aranui
50 Portsmouth Street
Wainoni Christchurch NZ
(03) 880 288

Natural Family Planning Centres:
276 Pitt Street
Sydney NSW 2000
(02) 890 5100

Catholic Family Planning Centre
371 Church Street
Richmond Vic 3121
(03) 9427 1233
Australia wide: (008) 33 3190
Country Victoria: (008) 11 4010

Centacare
Morgan Street
Fortitude Valley
Qld 4006
(07) 3252 4371

Centacare
33 Wakefield Street
Adelaide SA 5000
(08) 210 8200
1800 81 2300 (country areas)

Centacare Marriage & Family Service
456 Hay Street
Perth WA 6000
(09) 325 6644

Centacare
23 Stoke Street
New Town Tas 7008
(002) 78 1660

34 Francis Street
Rapid Creek NT 0810
(089) 85 1540

Natural Family Planning Centacare
42 Canberra Avenue
Forrest ACT 2603
(062) 239 7700

New Zealand Association of Natural Family Planning (Inc.)
PO Box 36-329
Northcote Auckland NZ
(09) 379 0184

PREGNANCY SUPPORT
See also Family Planning Association (under 'Contraceptive Advice') and 'Women's Health Centres'

Pregnancy Help
2 Alfred Road
Brookvale NSW 2100
(02) 9905 1974

Pregnancy Support
41 Park Street
Moonee Ponds Vic 3039
(03) 9370 3933

Pregnancy Help Brisbane, Inc.
7th Floor
201 Edward Street
Brisbane Qld 4000
(07) 3831 6161
(008) 77 7690 (outside Brisbane)

Spark Resource Centre (SA)
930 Port Road
Woodville West SA 5001
(08) 347 1109

Pregnancy Help
456 Hay Street
Perth WA 6000
(09) 325 5592

Pregnancy Support (Tas)
(002) 24 2290

Pregnancy Support (ACT)
(062) 49 1779

SUPPORT SERVICES — AUSTRALIA AND NEW ZEALAND

Pregnancy Help
18 Geranium Street
Stuart Park NT 0820
(089) 81 8526

Pregnancy Help
138 Queen Street
Auckland NZ
(04) 373 2599 (24 hours)

Pregnancy Counselling
 Services National Office
PO Box 33 432
Takapuna Auckland NZ
(09) 389 7271
(09) 307 6945 (24-hour
 counselling line)

Pregnancy Counselling
 Services
Wellington NZ
(04) 388 2831
(04) 383 5524 (counselling
 line)

WOMEN'S HEALTH CENTRES
See also Family Planning Association, under 'Contraceptive Advice'

Department for Women
Level 11
100 William Street
Darlinghurst NSW 2011
(02) 9334 1160
(008) 81 7227 (general
 information)

Leichhardt Women's Health
 Centre
55 Thornley Street
Leichhardt NSW 2040
(02) 560 3011

Liverpool Women's
 Community Health Centre
26 Bathurst Street
Liverpool NSW 2170
(02) 601 3555

Women's Information and
 Referral Exchange
1st Floor
Ross House
247 Flinders Lane
Melbourne Vic 3000
(03) 9654 6844
(008) 136 570
(9 a.m. to 7 p.m.)

Royal Women's Hospital
Bowen Bridge Road
Herston Qld 4029
(07) 3253 8111

Women's Infolink
Pavilion Building
Cnr Queen & Albert Streets
Brisbane Qld 4000
(07) 3229 1580
1 800 177 577

Women's Information
 Switchboard (SA)
(08) 223 1244
(008) 188 158

Women's Information and
 Referral Exchange
32 St Georges Terrace
Perth WA 6000
(09) 222 0444

Women's Health Care
 House
100 Aberdeen Street
Northbridge WA 6003
(09) 227 8122

Women's Information
 Service
GPO Box 1854
Hobart Tas 7000
(002) 34 2166

Hobart Women's Health
 Collective
GPO Box 1053
Hobart Tas 7000

Women's Information
 Centre
PO Box 721
Alice Springs NT 0871
(089) 51 5880

Women's Information and
 Referral Centre
Ground Floor
North Building
London Circuit
Canberra City ACT 2601
(06) 205 1075

National Women's Hospital
Claude Road
Auckland 3 NZ
(09) 638 9909

Christchurch Women's
 Hospital
885 Colombo Street
Christchurch NZ
(03) 364 4699

DOMESTIC VIOLENCE
Domestic Violence
 Counselling and Advice
1800 047 727 (24-hour free
 call, NSW only)

Domestic Violence and
 Incest Resource Centre
 (Vic)
(03) 387 9155

APPENDICES

Domestic Violence
Resource Centre
PO Box 3278
Sth Brisbane Qld 4101
(07) 3217 2344
(counselling and support)

Domestic Violence
Resource Unit
PO Box 39
Rundle Mall Post Office
Adelaide SA 5000
(08) 226 7065

Sexual and Domestic
Violence Crisis Care Unit
Adelaide SA
1800 800 098 (mobile
counselling and support)

Relationships Australia
755 Albany Highway
East Victoria Park WA 6100
(09) 470 5109

Crisis Care Unit (WA)
Metropolitan (09) 325 1111
Country (008) 199 008

Waratah Women's Support
Centre
PO Box 644
Bunbury WA 6230
(097) 91 2885

Family & Children's
Services (WA)
(09) 221 2000 (24-hour
family help line)
(008) 64 3000

Domestic Violence Crisis
Service (Tas.)
(002) 33 2529 (only
operates until midnight)
(002) 30 2111 (Police, for
calls received after
midnight)
1800 63 3937 (freecall
statewide)

Women's Shelter (Dawn
House)
Casuarina NT 0810
(089) 451 388

ACT Domestic Violence
Telephone and Information
Referral Service
(06) 248 7800 (24 hours)

Domestic Violence Support
Line
PO Box 106 126
Auckland NZ
(09) 303 3938
(09) 303 3939 (24-hour
support line)

Wellington Women's
Refuge
Wellington NZ
(04) 473 6280 (office and
crisis line)

Maori Women's Refuge
(04) 383 4945
(04) 389 2912 (crisis line)

Battered Women's Support
Group
Christchurch NZ
(03) 364 8900

WOMEN'S REFUGES
Women's Refuges NSW
(24-hour counselling
service)
(02) 560 1605

Homeless Persons
Information Centre (NSW)
(02) 265 9081

Women's Domestic
Violence Crisis Service
(Vic)
(03) 9329 8433 (24 hour)
1800 015 188 (country Vic)

Domestic Violence Hotline
(Qld)
Refuge Referral Line
(07) 384 4009

Sunnybank Family Support
Inc. (Qld)
(07) 345 6088

Emergency Housing Office
(SA)
(08) 207 0000

Domestic Violence
Outreach Service (SA)
(08) 267 4830 9 a.m.–4 p.m.

Women's Refuge
Multicultural Service (WA)
(09) 325 7716

Hobart Women's Shelter
(Tas)
(002) 34 6323

St Joseph's Child and
Family Support Centre
26 Channel Highway
Taroona Tas 7053
(002) 27 8705

Launceston Women's
Shelter (Tas)
(003) 34 3161

Ulverstone Women's
Shelter (Tas)
(004) 25 1382

SUPPORT SERVICES — AUSTRALIA AND NEW ZEALAND

Women's Shelter (Dawn
House)
Casuarina NT 0810
(089) 45 1388

Caroline Chisholm Women
& Children's Refuge
(ACT)
(06) 286 2173

Doris Women's Refuge
(ACT)
(06) 241 7028

Louisa Women's Refuge
Queanbeyan NSW 2620
(06) 299 4799

Wellington Women's
Refuge
Wellington NZ
(04) 73 6280
(04) 27 9212

RELATIONSHIPS AUST.
Relationships Australia
(NSW)
5 Sarah Street
Lane Cove NSW 2066
(02) 418 8800

Relationships Australia
(Vic)
46 Princess Street
Kew Vic 3101
(03) 9853 5354

Relationships Australia
159 St Paul's Terrace
Brisbane Qld 4000
(07) 3831 2005

Relationships Australia
(SA)
55 Hutt Street
Adelaide SA 5000
(08) 223 4566

Relatioships Australia (WA)
755 Albany Street
East Victoria Park WA 6101
(09) 470 5109

Centacare
306 Murray Street
Hobart TAS 7000
(002) 31 3141/31 4103

Relationships Australia
(NT)
Cnr Woods & Linsay Street
Darwin NT 0800
(089) 81 6676

Relationships Australia
(Canberra & Region)
15 Napier Close
Deakin ACT 2600
(06) 281 3600

Relationship Services Inc.
(NZ national office)
Ansett House
69–71 Boulcott Street
Wellington NZ
(09) 472 8798

**SINGLE OR LONE
PARENTS**
Parents Without Partners
Penrith NSW
(047) 30 2084

Lone Parents Family
Support Service
(Birthright)
Angel Place, 121 Pitt Street
Sydney NSW 2000
(02) 9232 6455
(02) 9232 6550

Parents Without Partners
PO Box 21
Canterbury Vic 3126
(03) 9836 3211

Council for Single Mothers
and Their Children
238 Flinders Lane
Melbourne Vic 3000
(03) 9415 1171

Parents Without Partners
Room 218 Gawler Place
Adelaide SA 5000
(08) 9232 3332

Lone Parents Family &
Support Service (SA)
(08) 8262 8441

Spark Resource Centre
(SA)
(08) 8347 1109

Parents Without Partners
Oasis Lotteries House
37 Hampden Road
Nedlands WA 6009
(09) 389 8350

Parents Without Partners
Hampson House
Hampton Road
Hobart Tas 7000
(002) 24 0893

Parents Without Partners
PO Box 465
Dickson ACT 2601
(06) 248 6333

Lone Fathers Association
(ACT)
(06) 258 4216

Birthright
Wellington NZ
(04) 72 0251
(04) 84 7966

APPENDICES

ABORIGINAL MEDICAL AND SUPPORT SERVICES
Aboriginal Medical Service
36 Turner Street
Redfern NSW 2016
(02) 9319 5823

Aboriginal Health Service
186 Nicholson Street
Fitzroy Vic 3065
(03) 9419 3000

Aboriginal and Islander Community Health Service
10 Hubert Street
Woolloongabba Qld 4102
(07) 3393 0055

Nunkuwarrin Yunti
182–190 Wakefield Street
Adelaide SA 5000
(08) 8223 5011

Aboriginal Medical Service
154 Edward Street
East Perth WA 6004
(09) 328 3888

Gloria Brennan Aboriginal Women's Information Centre (WA)
(09) 227 7097

Aboriginal Centre
198 Elizabeth Street
Hobart Tas 7000
(002) 34 8311

Aboriginal Women's Resource Centre
74 Smith Street
Darwin NT 0800
(089) 81 9601

CHILDCARE
Check in your local phone book under Early Childhood Health centres, Infant Welfare Centres or Plunket Nurses for the nearest centre.

Playgroups
Playgroup Association of NSW
145 Wellington Road
Sefton NSW 2162
(02) 9644 9066

Victorian Playgroup Association
346 Albert Street
Brunswick Vic 3056
(03) 9388 1599

Playgroup Association of Qld
396 Milton Road
Auchenflower Qld 4066
(07) 3371 8253

Playgroup Association of South Australia
47 Manton Street
Hindmarsh SA 5007
(08) 8346 2722

Playgroup Association of Western Australia
35 Wickham Street
East Perth WA 6004
(09) 221 3142

Playgroup Association of Tasmania
82 Hampden Road
Battery Point Tas 7000
(002) 23 4814

Playgroup Association of the Northern Territory
18 Bauhinia Street
Nightcliff NT 0810
(089) 85 4968

Playgroup Association Inc.
Former North Curtin primary School
Storey Street
Curtin ACT 2605
(06) 285 4336

POISONS INFORMATION SERVICES
AUSTRALIA-WIDE NUMBER: 131126

FIRST AID COURSES (ST JOHN AMBULANCE ASSOCIATION)
St John Ambulance Association
6 Hunt Street
Sydney NSW 2000
(02) 9212 1088

St John Ambulance Association
98 York Street
South Melbourne Vic 3000
(03) 9696 0390

St John Ambulance Association
225 St Paul's Terrace
Fortitude Valley Qld 4006
(07) 3252 3450

St John Ambulance Association
216 Greenhill Road
Eastwood SA 5063
(08) 8274 0444

SUPPORT SERVICES — AUSTRALIA AND NEW ZEALAND

St John Ambulance Association
209 Great Eastern Highway
Belmont WA 6104
(09) 277 9999

St John Ambulance Association
65 Fitzroy Crescent
South Hobart Tas 7000
(002) 23 7177

St John Ambulance Association
50 Dripstone Road
Casuarina NT 0810
(089) 22 6200

St John Ambulance Association
PO Box 3275
Manuka ACT 2603
(06) 295 3777

St John Ambulance Association
Cnr Marion and Vivian Streets
Wellington NZ
(04) 73 1315

CHILD ABUSE
If you are afraid that you might harm your baby, ring one of the following. These services can help you obtain support from other community agencies.

Child Protection and Family Crisis
Department of Community Services
(02) 9360 7200
088 06677 (Metropolitan & Country NSW)

Child Abuse Prevention Service (CAPS)
13 Norton Street
Ashfield NSW 2131
(02) 9716 8000 (24 hours)

Child Protection Unit
Health & Community Services (Vic)
(03) 9616 7777

Child Protection Unit
Royal Children's Hospital (Vic)
(03) 9345 5522

Parents Anonymous (Vic)
(03) 9654 4654 (7.00 a.m. to midnight)

Department of Family, Aboriginal and Islander Affairs
PO Box 806
Brisbane Qld 4001
(07) 3227 7111

Crisis Centre (Qld)
1800 17 7135

Community Awareness Unit
Queensland Centre for the Prevention of Child Abuse
(07) 3224 7588

Adelaide Children's Hospital
King William Road
North Adelaide SA 5006
(08) 8204 7000

Community Welfare Crisis Care Unit (SA)
(08) 813 1611

Department for Community Development (WA)
(09) 222 2555

Parent Help Centre
28 Alvan Street
Mt Lawley WA 6050
(09) 272 1466 (24-hour service)

Crisis Care (WA)
(09) 32 5111
(008) 19 9008

Child Protection Assessment Board
5th Floor
Kirksway House
2 Kirksway Place
Battery Point Tas 7004
(002) 33 2921 (24 hours)

Crisis Intervention Unit (Tas)
(002) 33 2529

Child & Family Protective Services (NT)
(089) 89 3939
(089) 41 1644 (after hours)

Child Protection Unit (ACT)
Northern Regional Office
(06) 207 1069
Southern Regional Office
(06) 207 1466
After hours (06) 295 1600

Parents Support Service (ACT)
(06) 247 0519

The New Zealand Child Abuse Prevention Society, Inc.
(24-hour services):

New Zealand Child Abuse Prevention Society
c/- Parent Help
PO Box 90217
Auckland NZ
(09) 579 0626

APPENDICES

Parent Help/Barnados
2 Edwin Street
Auckland NZ
(09) 638 8935
Counselling Line (09) 276 3311 (9 a.m.–3 p.m. Mon–Fri)

Parentline (Inc)
Box 11077
Hamilton NZ
(07) 839 4536

Parentline Hawkes Bay Inc.
Box 27
Hastings NZ
(06) 876 3658 (24 hours)

Parentline
Box 2014
Palmerston North (Manawatu) NZ
(06) 356 2679 (9 a.m.–12 p.m.)

Parentline
Box 395
Thames NZ
(843) 88 644

Parent Support Services (Wanganui Inc.)
Box 4347
Wanganui NZ
(06) 345 5331

Parentline
Box 28015
Kelburn (Wellington) NZ
(04) 499 9994

Norhtland
Box 5012
Regent (Whangarei) NZ
(09) 438 2151

COT DEATH/SUDDEN INFANT DEATH SUPPORT GROUPS

Sudden Infant Death Association
PO Box 2307
North Parramatta NSW 2151
(02) 630 0099
1800 65 1186 (24 hours)

National SIDS Council of Australia
357 Burwood Road
Hawthorn Vic 3122
(03) 9819 9277

Sudden Infant Death Research Foundation
1227 Malvern Road
Malvern Vic 3144
(03) 9822 9611

Sudden Infant Death Syndrome Parents' Network
PO Box 3388
South Brisbane Qld 4101
(07) 3899 2612

Queensland Sudden Infant Death Syndrome Foundation
PO Box 241
Mt Gravatt Qld 4122
(07) 3849 7122

SIDS Association of South Australia
301 Payneham Road
Royston Park SA 5070
(08) 363 1963

SIDS Foundation
33 Sixth Avenue
Kensington WA 6151
(09) 474 3544

Tasmanian SIDS Society, Inc.
PO Box 1007
Burnie Tas 7320
(004) 31 9488

SIDS Association of Northern Territory Inc.
PO Box 314
Sanderson NT 0812
Phone & Fax: (089) 27 2923

Sudden Infant Death Association
PO Box 887
Civic Square ACT 2608
(06 257 5164

New Zealand Cot Death Association
PO Box 28-177
Auckland NZ
(09) 524 8597

SIDS Canterbury Inc.
PO Box 13-620
Armagh, Christchurch NZ
(03) 364 8747

Otago Cot Death Society
PO Box 1709
Dunedin NZ
(024) 77 5025

BEREAVEMENT
(Stillbirth and Neonatal Death Support—SANDS)

NSW	(02) 906 7004
Vic	(03) 9882 1590
Qld	(07) 3252 2865
SA	(08) 277 0304
WA	(09) 382 2687
Tas	(004) 26 1137

NZ Bereaved Parents Group
(09) 58 6031

APPENDIX III

Immunisation schedules

Immunisation schedule for Australia

(National Health and Medical Research Council Standards Childhood Vaccination Schedule, August 1994)

Remember to keep a record of your baby's immunisation schedule.

2 months
First Triple Antigen for diphtheria, tetanus and whooping cough (pertussis), and oral Sabin for poliomyelitis and Haemophilus Influenza Type B (Hib)

4 months
Second Triple Antigen for diphtheria, tetanus and whooping cough (pertussis), and second oral Sabin for poliomyelitis and Haemophilus Influenza Type B (Hib)

6 months
Third Triple Antigen for diphtheria, tetanus and whooping cough (pertussis), and third oral Sabin for poliomyelitis Haemophilus Influenza Type B (Hib)

12 to 15 months
Combined measles, mumps and rubella injection

18 months
Fourth Triple Antigen for diphtheria, tetanus and whooping cough (pertussis) and Haemophilus Influenza Type B (Hib)

Prior to school entry (4–5 years)
Fifth Triple Antigen for diphtheria, tetanus and whooping cough (pertussis), and oral Sabin for poliomyelitis

10–16 years
Measles, mumps and rubella injection

15 years
Booster adult diphtheria and tetanus and oral Sabin

Further immunisations
Continue with tetanus immunisation every ten years.

Hepatitis B

Hepatitis B vaccine is given to babies whose parents are carriers or who come from a community known to have a high number of carriers. See page 91 for details. The schedule for hepatitis B is as follows:

Birth
Injection of Special Immune Globulin (if mother is a carrier) and first hepatitis B vaccine

1–2 months
Second hepatitis B vaccine

6 months
Third hepatitis B vaccine

The hepatitis B vaccines at two and six months can be given simultaneously with the Triple Antigen vaccine, but should be injected in different sites.

Tuberculosis

Tuberculosis immunisation is given to babies whose parents come from a country where there is a high incidence of tuberculosis. See page 91 for details. A BCG injection is given at birth.

Immunisation schedule for New Zealand
(to commence February 1996)
(Department of Health, New Zealand)

Newborn
Immunoglobulin injection for babies whose mothers are carriers of Hepatitis B

6 weeks
First Triple Antigen for diphtheria, tetanus and whooping cough (pertussis), and oral Sabin for poliomyelitis, and Hepatitis B vaccine and Haemophilus Influenza Type B (Hib)

3 months
Second Triple Antigen for diphtheria, tetanus and whooping cough (pertussis), and second oral Sabin for poliomyelitis, and Hepatitis B vaccine and Haemophilus Influenza Type B (Hib)

5 months
Third Triple Antigen for diphtheria, tetanus and whooping cough (pertussis), and third oral Sabin for poliomyelitis, and Hepatitis B vaccine and Haemophilus Influenza Type B (Hib)

15 months
Fourth Triple Antigen for diptheria, tetanus and whooping cough (pertussis), and Haemophilus Influenza Type B (Hib) and measles, mumps and rubella injection

11 years
Tetanus and diptheria injection, and fourth oral Sabin for poliomyelitis and second measles, mumps and rubella injection

Further immunisations
Tuberculosis immunisation is given at birth in some areas.

Tetanus immunisation is repeated after some injuries.

APPENDIX IV

Emergency Treatment

Choking

- Gently remove with your fingers any obvious obstruction, mucus or vomit.
- Place your baby across your lap, face down.
- Give two light blows with the heel of your hand between the baby's shoulder blades.
- If this fails, put your hands on either side of the baby's chest and give two sharp pushes inwards with a 2–3 second interval between the pushes.
- Call for an ambulance if you are unable to clear the airway immediately.
- If your baby's breathing is noisy, or she is unable to cry or is coughing, call an ambulance or go at once to your nearest hospital or doctor.

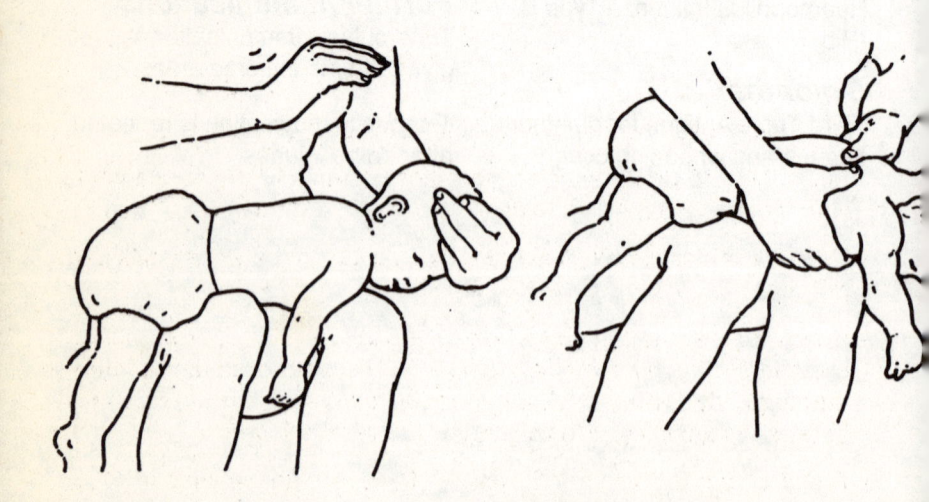

EMERGENCY TREATMENT

Resuscitation

If possible, send *someone else* to ring an ambulance (in **Australia dial 000**, in **New Zealand, 111**) and commence resuscitation yourself:

- Check the airway for blockages by first turning the baby's head to one side, then opening the mouth and looking inside.
- Gently remove any mucus or vomit with your fingers.
- Recheck breathing.
- If the baby is still not breathing, tilt her head back **slightly (diagram 1).**

1.

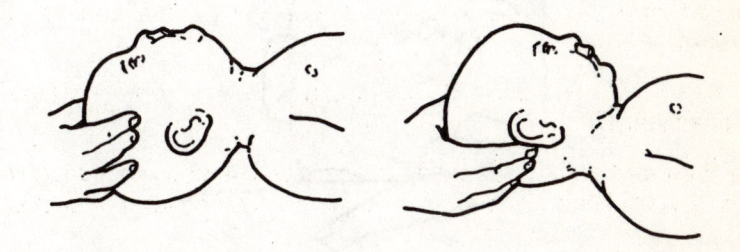

- Cover her nose and mouth with your own mouth **(diagram 2)**.
- Puff softly and slowly, watching the chest to see that it rises. Remove your mouth and let the air escape.
- Repeat the last two steps every three seconds **(twenty breaths per minute)**.
- Check for the brachial pulse beat **(diagram 3)**. If there is no pulse, place the baby on a hard, flat surface and commence **external heart massage (diagram 4)**. Compress the centre of the breastbone, between the nipples, with your index and middle fingers.
- Press down 1.5 cm to 2.5 cm ($1/2$–1") every half a second **(100 compressions per minute)**.

APPENDICES

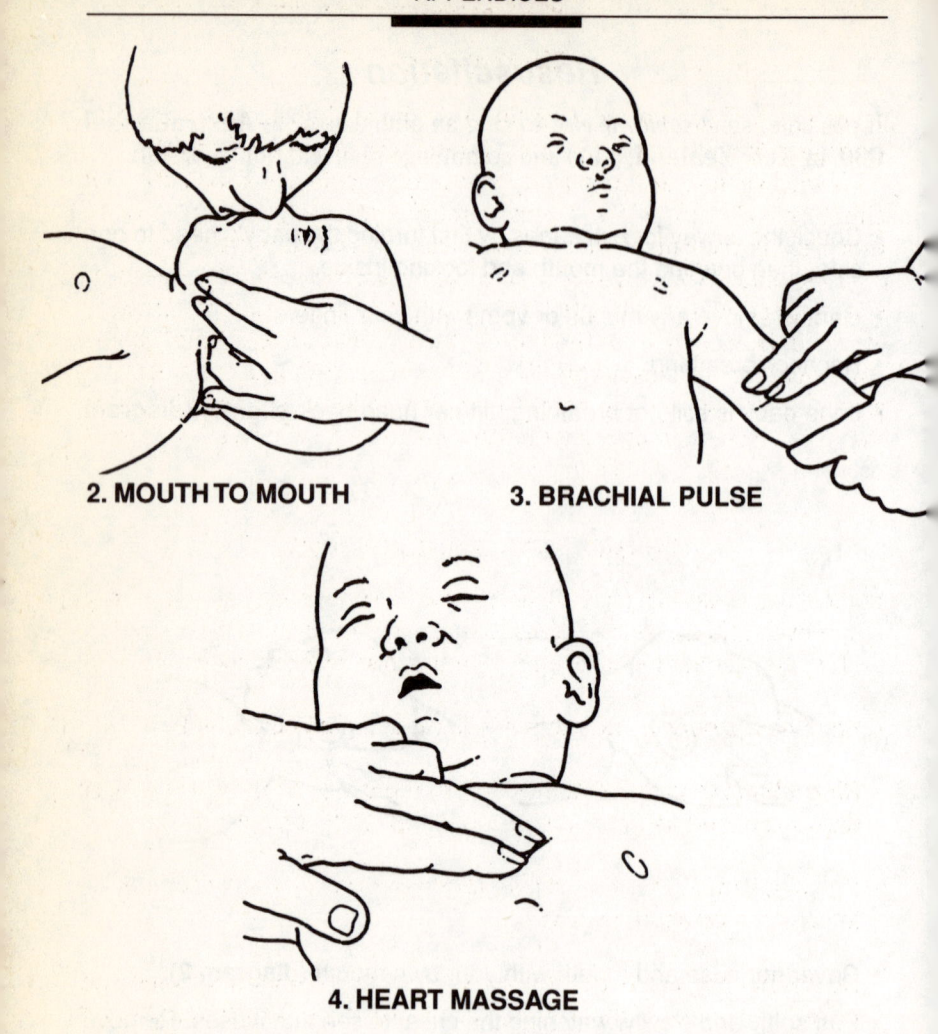

2. MOUTH TO MOUTH

3. BRACHIAL PULSE

4. HEART MASSAGE

- If you are alone with the baby, give her two breaths every fifteen compressions. If there are two people, have the other person give one breath every five compressions.

- Pause to recheck pulse and breathing after every minute of compressions. Once you can feel a pulse, do not continue with external heart massage.

- **Do not stop mouth-to-mouth resuscitation until the baby is breathing, or external heart massage until the baby has a pulse or help arrives.**

Tick bites

Some types of tick can be harmful to children. Their bite can bring on breathing difficulties, paralysis and drowsiness, but is rarely fatal.

If you live in an area of bush or you take your child bushwalking, you should check yourself and your children carefully for ticks. Look especially in the hair, behind or in the ears and near the anus.

Ticks should be removed whole, using sharp-pointed tweezers or scissors and levering the tick out gently to ensure that the head is attached. Do not squeeze the body of the tick as you remove it, as you will release more poison into the child. Unless it is in a very delicate area, use kerosene or mineral turpentine to kill the tick before you remove it. Have your baby checked by a doctor or hospital if she is unwell or if you are concerned in any way.

Snake and spider bites

Some Australian snakes and the Sydney funnel-web spider, the tree funnel-web spider and the red-back spider, can cause fatal poisoning.

If your child has been bitten by a venomous snake or spider:

- Keep her as quiet as possible and immobilise the bitten limb.

- **Ring 000 (111 in New Zealand)** for emergency medical help. Your baby may need an anti-venene to counteract the poison.

- Do not attempt to suck out the venom or wash the area, and do not try to open the puncture wound.

- Do not bandage red-back spider bites, as the venom is injected just under the surface of the skin and can be released over a twelve-hour period. For all other bites, apply a wide, firm bandage around the limb, starting at the bite area. Bandage as much of the limb as possible. If you do not have a bandage, use any clean cloth and maintain pressure on the bite area.

- Watch for symptoms of shock, difficulties in breathing, cardiac arrest and unconsciousness; these can occur from fifteen minutes to two hours after the bite. Treat these symptoms following the instructions on pages 255–6.

Bee stings and ant bites

These can be painful but are not dangerous unless your child has an allergic reaction. Seek medical advice if you are at all concerned.

Scrape the sting from the wound with your fingernail or remove it with tweezers, being careful not to squeeze it, as this injects more poison into the flesh, and apply ice wrapped in a cloth. You can also make a paste with a soluble aspirin tablet and apply this to the wound.

Watch for severe swelling. If the bite is on your baby's face or throat, seek medical advice, as the swelling can affect her breathing.

Index

Aboriginal medical and support services 247
abrupt weaning 153–4
adopted babies 19, 55
advice, coping with 35–6
advisory services 241–50
after-pains 37
air travel 198–9
alcohol
   during pregnancy 18
   while breastfeeding 130
allergic reaction
   to cow's milk 169
   to foods 174
animals 53, 106, 238–9
ant bites 258
antenatal classes 17
Apgar score 88
apple puree (recipe) 185
apricot puree (recipe) 185
asthma 18

'baby blues' 79
baby gates 29, 115, 123, 233
baby health centre sisters 11
baby care equipment 22–33
back protection 57
backache 38
backpacks 29
baked custard (recipe) 190
bassinettes 23, 24
bathing a baby 95–8
bathing equipment 27
bathroom safety 229
beans (recipe) 189
bedroom safety 230–1
bee stings 258
bereavement support 217–8, 249–50
bibs 32
birth experience 46–7
birthmarks 87
bites, poisonous 257–8

biting 112, 149
blankets 24–5
boiling method of sterilisation 166
bonding 48
bootees 30–32, 232
boredom in babies 67, 68
bottlefeeding 26, 159–70
bottles and teats 164–6
'bottom shuffling' 121
bouncers 29
bouncinettes 29, 233
bowel motions, babies' 93, 111
bras, maternity 129
breast massage 138
breast pads 147
breast pumps 138
breast refusal 147–8, 153
breastfeeding 26, 126–58
   advice 241
   as a method of contraception 46
   with hospitalised mother or baby 50–1
breastmilk
   composition of 127–8
   expression of 131, 136–7, 137–8, 155–6
   increasing supply of 145–6
   leaking of 147
   oversupply of 146–7
   production of 127
   storage of 139
breasts care of 128–9
   during weaning 155–6
   engorgement of 143
broth (recipe) 187
burping 66

caesarean section 37–8
   breastfeeding after 135

camping holidays 195–6
Candida albicans, see thrush
canned baby food 180–1
capsules, safety 24, 194, 237–8
car safety 193–4, 237–8
car seats for babies 194, 237–8
caravan holidays 194–5
carry cots 23, 24
casein-based milks 160
cats 53, 239
cephalhaematoma 86
cereals 174
change tables and mats 25
changing nappies 94
   equipment for 25–6
cheese 175
cheese and potato patties (recipe) 188
chemical sterilisation of equipment 164–5
chicken 176
child abuse support groups 248–9
child minding 117
childbirth education classes 17
childcare 219–24, 247–8
childproofing your home 20–1, 115, 227–34
choking 254
circuit breakers 227
circumcision 22
classes, childbirth education 17
cleft palate 140
clothing for babies 29–32
   safety of 232
coach and train travel 196–8
coffee and tea intake while breastfeeding 130

259

colds, common 215–16
colic 68–9
colostrum 127, 128
comfort settling 119–20
commercial baby food 180
common colds 215–16
complementary feeds 134
condoms 45
constipation
  of baby 212
  post-natal 37
contraception 44–6
  advice on 243–4
contraceptive pills 44–5
cot death 217–18
  support groups 249–50
cots 23–4, 104
  portable 201–2
cotton tips 25
counselling service,
  Tresillian 10
counselling services 241–2
cow's milk 159–60
  allergic reaction to 169
cradle cap 215
crawling 121
creams, applying 206–7
crying babies 63–76
custard, baked (recipe) 190
cystic fibrosis 88, 89

Day Stay Clinics, Tresillian 10
daytime sleeps 108, 118–9
dehydration 93, 212, 237
  prevention of, while travelling 199
demand feeding 131
dental care 113–4
depression, post-natal, see post-natal depression
dermatitis, see cradle cap
developmental stages
  newborn 85
  three to six months 102
  six months 108
  nine months 116
  twelve months 116
diaphragms 45

diarrhoea 210–11
diet, balanced 173, 177
  while breastfeeding 130
dining and living area safety 229–30
dishwasher powder 228
disposable nappies 30, 194
dogs 53, 238–9
domestic violence support groups 245–6
door barriers 29, 115, 123, 233
dummies 26–7, 68, 103–4
  safety with 232

earache 217
early childhood health nurses 11
eggs 176
electric blankets 67
electrical appliance safety 68, 227, 228, 229, 230–1
emergency resuscitation 255–6
emergency phone numbers checklist 14
  support services 241–50
enhancing development 99, 105–6, 114–5, 121–2
episiotomy 37
equipment for baby care 22–33
equipment for travelling, see travelling
establishing breastfeeding 131–2
exercises
  post-natal 38–9, 40–1
  relaxation, for baby 72, 74–5
  relaxation, for parents 57
expectations of parenthood 11, 54–5, 78–9
expressing breastmilk 131, 136–9, 137–8, 155–6

fads in parenting 12
falls, avoiding 100, 107, 229, 233

Family Day Care 220
Family Planning Association 243–4
family planning 45
fast flow of breastmilk 146
feeding 126–90
  equipment 26
  from three months to six months 104–5
  from six to nine months 110
  from nine to twelve months 117
fevers 111, 207–9
finger foods 175–6
firearm safety 233-4
first aid, emergency 254–8
first aid classes 19, 204, 248
first aid kit 19, 123
  suggested contents 226–7
fish 175
  baked (recipe) 186–7
flat nipples 144-5
floor play 67, 99, 105, 114, 121
flouride 113, 179
flouride tablets while driving 201
fontanelles 86, 97
food additives 181
food labelling 181
foods to avoid 177–8
foremilk 128
formulas 160–63
frezzing and thawing food 179–80
fruit 174–5
  gel (recipe) 186
  puree (recipe) 185
fruit juice 178–9

galactosaemia 88, 89
games, 122
garage safety 234
garden safety 235–6
gastroenteritis 210, 211
gates, baby 29, 115, 123, 233
goat's milk 160–1
gradual weaning 153

INDEX

suggested timetable 154
group therapy for post-natal depression 82–3
gun safety 233–4
Guthrie Child Care Centre 10
Guthrie test 88

haemophilus influenzae type b (Hib) 90–1
hand expressing breastmilk 138–9
health problems in new babies 49–50
hearing problems 114
heart massage 256
heating formula 163
hepatitis B 99, 252
high temperature 207–9
highchairs 110, 230, 233
  portable 202
hindmilk 128
holidaying with a baby 192–202
home births 17
hospital births 17
hospitalised babies 49–50
hot weather, care of babies in 67, 92–3, 104
housework management 58–9
humanised formulas 160–1
hygiene with pets 238–9
hypothyroidism 88, 89

immunisation 89–91
  schedules 251–3
insufficient breastmilk 145–6
intra-uterine devices 45
introduction of solid food 171–83
  suggested sequence 179
inverted nipples 144–5
isolation of new parents 19–20
IUDs 45

jaundice 89

juices 178–9
junket (recipe) 188

kitchen safety 181–2, 228–9

lack of breastmilk 145–6
lack of sleep, parental 39, 42, 76
laundering nappies 94–5
laundry
  equipment 27–8
  safety 231
lead paint 23
leaking breastmilk 43, 147
legumes 177
  (recipe) 189
lentils (recipe) 189
'let-down reflex' 127
liquid formula 162
living and dining area safety 229–30
lochia 36–7
locks, childproof 227, 228
long day care 220
lotions, applying, 206–7
lowering a high temperature 207–9

marriage guidance 246–7
massage, baby 27, 70–2
mastitis 143–4
maternity bras 129
mattresses and mattress covers 24
mealtimes 182
measles 91
meat 176
meat broth (recipe) 187
medication
  during pregnancy 18–19
  for babies 204–5
  for teething 110–13
  for travel sickness 193
  in breastmilk 82, 131
medicines
  administering 205–6
  storing 229
microwave ovens
  cooking, see recipes 184–90

heating formula in 163
  heating food in 183
  safety 228
middle ear infection 217
milia 86
mittens 32, 232
Mongolian spots 87
monilia, see thrush
morning-after pill 46
mosquito nets 25
mothering role, expectations of 11, 54–5, 78–9
mouth-to-mouth resuscitation 255–6
muesli (recipe) 190
multiple births 32
  breastfeeding after 135–6
  support groups 247–8
mumps 91
music 69, 71, 115, 122
mutual weaning 153
myths
  about motherhood 78–9
  about weaning 152

nail cutting 95
nappies 29–30
  disposable 30, 194
  washing 94–5
nappy changing 94
  equipment 25–6
nappy liners 94
nappy rash 30, 68, 213
Natural Family Planning Centres 243–4
night clothes 30
night waking 102–4
nipple shields 144–5
nipples
  care of 129, 142
  flat or inverted 144–5
NMAA 140, 243
nursery
  equipment 23–6
  safety 231
Nursing Mothers' Association of Australia 140, 243
nuts 177

261

oatmeal porridge (recipe) 189
occasional care 220
oil, baby 27, 71
ointments, applying 206–7
older children and a new baby 21–2, 52
outdoor play equipment 235
Outreach Service, Tresillian 10
overseas travel 200–1
oversupply of breastmilk 167–7
overstimulation of baby 68
oxytocin 127

packaged foods 180
parenting role, expectations of 11, 54–5, 78–9
pear puree (recipe) 185
pets 53, 238–9
phenylketonuria 88, 89
physical changes, post-natal 36–8
pilchers 30
pillows 24
plastic pants 30
play equipment
  outdoor 235
  see also toys
playgroups 121, 247–8
playpens 28–9, 227, 229
Plunket nurses 11
poisonous plants and animals 236
poisons information 248
pool safety 234–5
porridge, oatmeal (recipe) 189
portable cots 201–2
portable highchairs 202
positioning for breastfeeding 132–3
positive attitude, maintenance of 55–7
post-natal depression 62, 78–84
  support groups 242
  Tresillian service 10

post-natal exercises 38–9, 40–1, 57
posture feeding 146
potato and cheese patties (recipe) 188
pouches, baby 29
powdered formula 160–1
prams and strollers 28, 233
pregnancy 16–19
  support groups 244
premature babies 48–9
  breastfeeding of 131, 136–7
pre-natal classes 17
preparing formula 161–3
prickly heat 92–3
problems with breastfeeding 141–50
prune juice (recipe) 185

quadruplets, see multiple births

rashes 111–2
recipes 184–90
red meat 176
refusal by babies
  of the bottle 155, 157–8
  of the breast 147–8, 153
  of solids 172
relationship, maintaining parents' 46–7, 83
relaxation
  bath for 72
  exercises, baby 72, 74–5
  techniques for parents 57
residential units, Tresillian 10
  addresses of 241
resuscitation 255–6
rice, creamed (recipe) 186
rubella 91
rugs 32
rusks (recipe) 190

Sabin, oral 90
safety measures 226–40
  for babies birth to three months 99

  for babies three to six months old 106
  for babies six to nine months old 115
  for babies nine to twelve months old 122–3
  in the bath 98
  in the bathroom 229
  in the bedroom 230–1
  in the car 99, 193–4, 237–8
  in the caravan 194–5
  in dining and living areas 229–30
  in the garden 235–6
  in the garage 234
  in the kitchen 181–2, 228–9
  in the laundry 231
  in the nursery 231
  near water 199–200, 234–5
  to prevent falls 990, 106, 233
  to prevent sunburn 236–7
  when cooking and feeding 182–3, 228–9
  when ironing 227
  when visiting 239
  with animals 53, 238–9
  with clothing 232
  with cots 103, 201–2
  with electrical appliances 67, 227, 228, 229, 230–1
  with firearms 233–4
  with food 176, 182–3
  with outdoor play equipment 235
  with toys 231–2
salt 177, 183
separation from baby or older child 50–1
settling babies 65–75, 119–20
sexual intercourse, post-natal 43–4
sheets, cot 24
shoes 120

INDEX

siblings 21–2, 52
sick babies
   breastfeeding 136–7
   caring for 203–18
SIDS, *see* Sudden Infant Death Syndrome
single parent support groups 247
six-week post-natal check 39
sleep, parental lack of 39–43, 76
sleep, baby's 64–5
   three to six months 102–4
   six to nine months 109
   nine to twelve months 118–9
sleepy bottlefed babies 168–9
smoking
   during pregnancy 18
   while breastfeeding 130
snake and spider bites 257
solid food, introduction of 104–, 170, 171–83
soup (recipe) 187
soya milk formulas 161
speech 120
steam sterilisers 166
sterilisation as a method of contraception 46
sterilising bottles and teats 164–5
sterilising solution for nappies 95
sticky eyes 92
Stillbirth and Neonatal Death Support 250
stimulating babies 99, 105–6, 114–5, 121–2
storing breastmilk 139–40
storing formula 162, 163
stork-marks 87
stove guards 228
straps, safety 233
strawberry marks 88
strollers and prams 28, 233
Sudden Infant Death Syndrome 217–18

support groups 249–50
sugar 113, 177, 183
sunburn 196, 199–200, 236–7
sunscreen 196, 236–7
supervision of children near water 234–5
support network, personal 20
support services 241–50
suppression of lactation 155–6
survival techniques for new parents 54–62, 73
swimming pool safety 234–5

taking a baby's temperature 208
tea and coffee intake while breastfeeding 130
teats and bottles 164–6
teeth, care of 113
teething 110–13
telephone numbers of support services 241–50
thawing frozen food 179–80
thrush 142–3, 214–15
tick bites 257
toddlers and a new baby 21–2, 52
tooth decay 113–14
toy libraries 122
toys
   safety of 231–2
   birth to three months 99
   three to six months 105
   six to nine months 114
   nine months to one year 122
train and coach travel 196–8
transporting formula 163
travelling 192–202
travel sickness medication 193
Tresillian Family Care Centres 9
Triple Antigen injections 90, 251, 253

triplets, *see* multiple births
tuberculosis 91, 252, 252

ultrasound scan 17–18
umbilical cord care 25, 87–8
unsettled babies 63–76, 149, 168–9
unwell babies, *see* sick babies
'use by' date
   food 181
   formula 163
   medication 205
uterus 36–37

vegetables 175
vegetarian diets 178
vomiting 209–10

waking at night 103–4
walkers, baby 29
walking 120
washing nappies 94–5
water beds 230
water, given to babies 66
water safety 199–200, 234–5
water travel 199–200
weaning 151–8
weight gain 134–5
   birth to three months 85
   three to six months 101
   six to nine months 108
   nine to twelve months 116
whey-based milks 161
wind 65–6
women's health centres 246–7
women's refuges 244
working mothers 222–4
   and bottlefeeding 168
   and breastfeeding 137–8
wrapping new babies 66

yoghurt 175
   (recipe) 188

Acknowledgements

To Brian, who is always there to share the joys and difficulties of parenting; my two sons Hugh and Martin, who have allowed me to revisit the magic years; my sister and lifelong friend Irene; our parents May and Jim, who have given love and support — CF

Thank you to my mother, Joyce, for teaching me her mothercraft skills and to my father Colin Gornall for his quiet support. To Maryanne, Jane, Lynne and John, who gave me first-hand knowledge of family life, and to their partners and children. To my friends who supported and encouraged me while this manuscript was being prepared — PG

Thank you to the members of the Tresillian Council for their ongoing support and especially Mrs Alison Cox, for the encouragement and advice she provided as the President of Tresillian at the time of the initial publication of this book.

Thank you to all the staff at Tresillian for support and encouragement, especially Mrs Pamela Fikar, Executive Director of Nursing, and the late Mr Clem Potter, Chief Executive Officer.

Thank you to Miss Evangelyn Carr and Mrs Anne Kulscar for their encouragement and for keeping the cogs of education turning while the manuscript was being written.

A special thank you to the nursing and medical staff, who read parts of the manuscript and gave valuable critical comment and clinical expertise: Karen Bowring, Penelope Field, Pamela McLennan, Elizabeth Nicolls, Anne Partridge, Beryl Rodionoff, Eva Stuhl and Mary Wickham; to social workers Rosemary Seale and Sue Williams for their assistance with the chapter on post-natal depression; to the nurses outside Tresillian who gave their time and their clinical expertise and comments Debra Lee and Margaret Guest from Belmore and Lakemba Early Childhood Health Centres and Gail Bryson from Armidale Area Health Centre; to Gloria Breneger from Walgett District Hospital for her advice and expertise on parenting in hot and isolated areas; to the parents and students, past and present, who have challenged our ideas and helped us grow personally and professionally; to Ann Paton for her public relations skills in the early conception of this book; to Margo Lanagan, Steven Dunbar, Jennifer Burns and Kirsty Melville for bringing this book together.

For all their help and support for the revised edition of this book we would like to thank: Neville Don (Directoe of Medical Services); Brenda Gillard (lactation consultant); David Hannaford (General Manager); and Florence Trout (Plunkett, New Zealand).